MIGRAINE
TRACKER

A chronic migraine journal & log book

Name/ Contact Details

_____

_____

_____

Emergency Contact

_____

_____

_____

Doctor/ Hospital Information

_____

_____

_____

_____

_____

_____

Migraine Log Overview - Page 1

Return to this page to log each of your migraine journal entries. (1-15)
Record the date, duration, pain level (low, moderate, severe) and notes, for each entry.

#	Date	Duration	Pain Level	Notes
1				
2				
3				
4				
5				
6				
7				
8				
9				
10				
11				
12				
13				
14				
15				

Notes

_____

_____

Migraine Log Overview - Page 2

Return to this page to log each of your migraine journal entries. (16-30)
Record the date, duration, pain level (low, moderate, severe) and notes, for each entry.

#	Date	Duration	Pain Level	Notes
16				
17				
18				
19				
20				
21				
22				
23				
24				
25				
26				
27				
28				
29				
30				

Notes

Migraine Log Overview - Page 3

Return to this page to log each of your migraine journal entries. (31-45)
Record the date, duration, pain level (low, moderate, severe) and notes, for each entry.

#	Date	Duration	Pain Level	Notes
31				
32				
33				
34				
35				
36				
37				
38				
39				
40				
41				
42				
43				
44				
45				

Notes

Migraine Log Overview - Page 4

Return to this page to log each of your migraine journal entries. (46-60)
Record the date, duration, pain level (low, moderate, severe) and notes, for each entry.

#	Date	Duration	Pain Level	Notes
46				
47				
48				
49				
50				
51				
52				
53				
54				
55				
56				
57				
58				
59				
60				

Notes

Entry #: _____ Date: _____ Duration: _____

Onset: ☐ Slow ☐ Average ☐ Rapid

Pain level: ☐ Mild ☐ Moderate ☐ Severe

Pain Location

(Mark with an "X")

Pain Description

☐ Throbbing ☐ Piercing ☐ Pounding

☐ Dull ☐ Burning ☐ Pulsating

☐ Constant ☐ Debilitating ☐ Squeezing

☐ Other _____

Left, right, center: _____

Symptoms

☐ Light sensitivity ☐ Sound sensitivity ☐ Aura ☐ Confusion

☐ Dizziness ☐ Nausea ☐ Vomiting ☐ Chills

☐ Muscle aches ☐ Muscle stiffness ☐ Restlessness ☐ Congestion

☐ Coughing ☐ Diarrhea ☐ Fever ☐ Sore throat

Other symptoms: _____

Health

Physical activity (past week): ☐ Low ☐ Moderate ☐ High

Sleep quality (past week): ☐ Poor ☐ Average ☐ Good

Computer time (past week): ☐ Low ☐ Moderate ☐ High

Stress level (past 3 days): ☐ Low ☐ Moderate ☐ High

Hormones

☐ PMS ☐ Menstruation ☐ Menopause ☐ Puberty ☐ Other: _____

Treatments Applied

Medication(s)/
dosage: _____

☐ Massage ☐ Stretching/ yoga ☐ Nerve stimulation device

☐ Heat/bath ☐ Acupuncture ☐ Ice packs

Other: _____

Weather/ Altitude

Temperature: _____   Humidity: _____   Barometric pressure: _____

Pollen level: ☐ Low   ☐ Moderate   ☐ High   Current elevation: _____

Food Tracking

	Today	Yesterday
Meals/ snacks:		

	Today	Yesterday
Vitamins/ supplements:		

	Today	Past 5 days
Alcoholic beverages:		
Caffeinated beverages:		
8oz glasses of water:		

Additional Notes

_____
_____
_____
_____
_____

Doctor's Notes

Dr. Name: _____   Specialty: _____   Date: _____

_____
_____
_____
_____
_____
_____

Entry #: _____ Date: _____ Duration: _____

Onset: ☐ Slow ☐ Average ☐ Rapid

Pain level: ☐ Mild ☐ Moderate ☐ Severe

Pain Location
(Mark with an "X")

Pain Description

☐ Throbbing ☐ Piercing ☐ Pounding

☐ Dull ☐ Burning ☐ Pulsating

☐ Constant ☐ Debilitating ☐ Squeezing

☐ Other _____

Left, right, center: _____

Symptoms

☐ Light sensitivity ☐ Sound sensitivity ☐ Aura ☐ Confusion

☐ Dizziness ☐ Nausea ☐ Vomiting ☐ Chills

☐ Muscle aches ☐ Muscle stiffness ☐ Restlessness ☐ Congestion

☐ Coughing ☐ Diarrhea ☐ Fever ☐ Sore throat

Other symptoms: _____

Health

Physical activity (past week): ☐ Low ☐ Moderate ☐ High

Sleep quality (past week): ☐ Poor ☐ Average ☐ Good

Computer time (past week): ☐ Low ☐ Moderate ☐ High

Stress level (past 3 days): ☐ Low ☐ Moderate ☐ High

Hormones

☐ PMS ☐ Menstruation ☐ Menopause ☐ Puberty ☐ Other: _____

Treatments Applied

Medication(s)/ dosage: _____

☐ Massage ☐ Stretching/ yoga ☐ Nerve stimulation device

☐ Heat/bath ☐ Acupuncture ☐ Ice packs

Other: _____

Weather/ Altitude

Temperature: Humidity: Barometric pressure:

Pollen level: ☐ Low   ☐ Moderate   ☐ High   Current elevation:

Food Tracking

	Today	Yesterday
Meals/ snacks:		

	Today	Yesterday
Vitamins/ supplements:		

	Today	Past 5 days
Alcoholic beverages:		
Caffeinated beverages:		
8oz glasses of water:		

Additional Notes

_____
_____
_____
_____
_____

Doctor's Notes

Dr. Name: _____ Specialty: _____ Date: _____

_____
_____
_____
_____
_____

Entry #: _____ Date: _____ Duration: _____

Onset: ☐ Slow ☐ Average ☐ Rapid

Pain level: ☐ Mild ☐ Moderate ☐ Severe

Pain Location
(Mark with an "X")

Pain Description

☐ Throbbing ☐ Piercing ☐ Pounding

☐ Dull ☐ Burning ☐ Pulsating

☐ Constant ☐ Debilitating ☐ Squeezing

☐ Other _____

Left, right, center: _____

Symptoms

☐ Light sensitivity ☐ Sound sensitivity ☐ Aura ☐ Confusion

☐ Dizziness ☐ Nausea ☐ Vomiting ☐ Chills

☐ Muscle aches ☐ Muscle stiffness ☐ Restlessness ☐ Congestion

☐ Coughing ☐ Diarrhea ☐ Fever ☐ Sore throat

Other symptoms: _____

Health

Physical activity (past week): ☐ Low ☐ Moderate ☐ High

Sleep quality (past week): ☐ Poor ☐ Average ☐ Good

Computer time (past week): ☐ Low ☐ Moderate ☐ High

Stress level (past 3 days): ☐ Low ☐ Moderate ☐ High

Hormones

☐ PMS ☐ Menstruation ☐ Menopause ☐ Puberty ☐ Other: _____

Treatments Applied

Medication(s)/ dosage: _____

☐ Massage ☐ Stretching/ yoga ☐ Nerve stimulation device

☐ Heat/bath ☐ Acupuncture ☐ Ice packs

Other: _____

Weather/ Altitude

Temperature: _____   Humidity: _____   Barometric pressure: _____

Pollen level: ☐ Low ☐ Moderate ☐ High   Current elevation: _____

Food Tracking

	Today	Yesterday
Meals/ snacks:		

	Today	Yesterday
Vitamins/ supplements:		

	Today	Past 5 days
Alcoholic beverages:		
Caffeinated beverages:		
8oz glasses of water:		

Additional Notes

_____

_____

_____

_____

_____

Doctor's Notes

Dr. Name: _____ Specialty: _____ Date: _____

_____

_____

_____

_____

_____

_____

Entry #: _____ Date: _____ Duration: _____

Onset: ☐ Slow ☐ Average ☐ Rapid

Pain level: ☐ Mild ☐ Moderate ☐ Severe

Pain Location
(Mark with an "X")

Pain Description

☐ Throbbing ☐ Piercing ☐ Pounding

☐ Dull ☐ Burning ☐ Pulsating

☐ Constant ☐ Debilitating ☐ Squeezing

☐ Other _____

Left, right, center: _____

Symptoms

☐ Light sensitivity ☐ Sound sensitivity ☐ Aura ☐ Confusion

☐ Dizziness ☐ Nausea ☐ Vomiting ☐ Chills

☐ Muscle aches ☐ Muscle stiffness ☐ Restlessness ☐ Congestion

☐ Coughing ☐ Diarrhea ☐ Fever ☐ Sore throat

Other symptoms: _____

Health

Physical activity (past week): ☐ Low ☐ Moderate ☐ High

Sleep quality (past week): ☐ Poor ☐ Average ☐ Good

Computer time (past week): ☐ Low ☐ Moderate ☐ High

Stress level (past 3 days): ☐ Low ☐ Moderate ☐ High

Hormones

☐ PMS ☐ Menstruation ☐ Menopause ☐ Puberty ☐ Other: _____

Treatments Applied

Medication(s)/ dosage: _____

☐ Massage ☐ Stretching/ yoga ☐ Nerve stimulation device

☐ Heat/bath ☐ Acupuncture ☐ Ice packs

Other: _____

Weather/ Altitude

Temperature: _____   Humidity: _____   Barometric pressure: _____

Pollen level: ◯ Low   ◯ Moderate   ◯ High   Current elevation: _____

Food Tracking

	Today	Yesterday
Meals/ snacks:		

	Today	Yesterday
Vitamins/ supplements:		

	Today	Past 5 days
Alcoholic beverages:		
Caffeinated beverages:		
8oz glasses of water:		

Additional Notes

_____
_____
_____
_____
_____

Doctor's Notes

Dr. Name: _____ Specialty: _____ Date: _____

_____
_____
_____
_____
_____
_____

Entry #: _____ Date: _____ Duration: _____

Onset: ☐ Slow ☐ Average ☐ Rapid

Pain level: ☐ Mild ☐ Moderate ☐ Severe

Pain Location
(Mark with an "X")

Left, right, center: _____

Pain Description

☐ Throbbing ☐ Piercing ☐ Pounding

☐ Dull ☐ Burning ☐ Pulsating

☐ Constant ☐ Debilitating ☐ Squeezing

☐ Other _____

Symptoms

☐ Light sensitivity ☐ Sound sensitivity ☐ Aura ☐ Confusion

☐ Dizziness ☐ Nausea ☐ Vomiting ☐ Chills

☐ Muscle aches ☐ Muscle stiffness ☐ Restlessness ☐ Congestion

☐ Coughing ☐ Diarrhea ☐ Fever ☐ Sore throat

Other symptoms: _____

Health

Physical activity (past week): ☐ Low ☐ Moderate ☐ High

Sleep quality (past week): ☐ Poor ☐ Average ☐ Good

Computer time (past week): ☐ Low ☐ Moderate ☐ High

Stress level (past 3 days): ☐ Low ☐ Moderate ☐ High

Hormones

☐ PMS ☐ Menstruation ☐ Menopause ☐ Puberty ☐ Other: _____

Treatments Applied

Medication(s)/dosage: _____

☐ Massage ☐ Stretching/ yoga ☐ Nerve stimulation device

☐ Heat/bath ☐ Acupuncture ☐ Ice packs

Other: _____

Weather/ Altitude

Temperature: Humidity: Barometric pressure:

Pollen level: ☐ Low   ☐ Moderate   ☐ High   Current elevation:

Food Tracking

	Today	Yesterday
Meals/ snacks:		

	Today	Yesterday
Vitamins/ supplements:		

	Today	Past 5 days
Alcoholic beverages:		
Caffeinated beverages:		
8oz glasses of water:		

Additional Notes

_____
_____
_____
_____
_____

Doctor's Notes

Dr. Name: _____ Specialty: _____ Date: _____

_____
_____
_____
_____
_____
_____

Entry #: _____ Date: _____ Duration: _____

Onset: ◻ Slow ◻ Average ◻ Rapid

Pain level: ◻ Mild ◻ Moderate ◻ Severe

Pain Location
(Mark with an "X")

Pain Description

◻ Throbbing ◻ Piercing ◻ Pounding

◻ Dull ◻ Burning ◻ Pulsating

◻ Constant ◻ Debilitating ◻ Squeezing

◻ Other _____

Left, right, center: _____

Symptoms

◻ Light sensitivity ◻ Sound sensitivity ◻ Aura ◻ Confusion

◻ Dizziness ◻ Nausea ◻ Vomiting ◻ Chills

◻ Muscle aches ◻ Muscle stiffness ◻ Restlessness ◻ Congestion

◻ Coughing ◻ Diarrhea ◻ Fever ◻ Sore throat

Other symptoms: _____

Health

Physical activity (past week): ◻ Low ◻ Moderate ◻ High

Sleep quality (past week): ◻ Poor ◻ Average ◻ Good

Computer time (past week): ◻ Low ◻ Moderate ◻ High

Stress level (past 3 days): ◻ Low ◻ Moderate ◻ High

Hormones

◻ PMS ◻ Menstruation ◻ Menopause ◻ Puberty ◻ Other: _____

Treatments Applied

Medication(s)/ dosage: _____

◻ Massage ◻ Stretching/ yoga ◻ Nerve stimulation device

◻ Heat/bath ◻ Acupuncture ◻ Ice packs

Other: _____

Weather/ Altitude

Temperature: _____   Humidity: _____   Barometric pressure: _____

Pollen level: ☐ Low   ☐ Moderate   ☐ High   Current elevation: _____

Food Tracking

	Today	Yesterday
Meals/ snacks:		

	Today	Yesterday
Vitamins/ supplements:		

	Today	Past 5 days
Alcoholic beverages:		
Caffeinated beverages:		
8oz glasses of water:		

Additional Notes

_____
_____
_____
_____
_____

Doctor's Notes

Dr. Name: _____ Specialty: _____ Date: _____

_____
_____
_____
_____
_____
_____

Entry #: _____ Date: _____ Duration: _____

Onset: ☐ Slow ☐ Average ☐ Rapid

Pain level: ☐ Mild ☐ Moderate ☐ Severe

Pain Location
(Mark with an "X")

Pain Description

☐ Throbbing ☐ Piercing ☐ Pounding

☐ Dull ☐ Burning ☐ Pulsating

☐ Constant ☐ Debilitating ☐ Squeezing

☐ Other _____

Left, right, center: _____

Symptoms

☐ Light sensitivity ☐ Sound sensitivity ☐ Aura ☐ Confusion

☐ Dizziness ☐ Nausea ☐ Vomiting ☐ Chills

☐ Muscle aches ☐ Muscle stiffness ☐ Restlessness ☐ Congestion

☐ Coughing ☐ Diarrhea ☐ Fever ☐ Sore throat

Other symptoms: _____

Health

Physical activity (past week): ☐ Low ☐ Moderate ☐ High

Sleep quality (past week): ☐ Poor ☐ Average ☐ Good

Computer time (past week): ☐ Low ☐ Moderate ☐ High

Stress level (past 3 days): ☐ Low ☐ Moderate ☐ High

Hormones

☐ PMS ☐ Menstruation ☐ Menopause ☐ Puberty ☐ Other: _____

Treatments Applied

Medication(s)/ dosage: _____

☐ Massage ☐ Stretching/ yoga ☐ Nerve stimulation device

☐ Heat/bath ☐ Acupuncture ☐ Ice packs

Other: _____

Weather/ Altitude

Temperature: _____   Humidity: _____   Barometric pressure: _____

Pollen level: ☐ Low   ☐ Moderate   ☐ High   Current elevation: _____

Food Tracking

	Today	Yesterday
Meals/ snacks:		

	Today	Yesterday
Vitamins/ supplements:		

	Today	Past 5 days
Alcoholic beverages:		
Caffeinated beverages:		
8oz glasses of water:		

Additional Notes

_____
_____
_____
_____
_____

Doctor's Notes

Dr. Name: _____   Specialty: _____   Date: _____

_____
_____
_____
_____
_____
_____

Entry #: _____ Date: _____ Duration: _____

Onset: ☐ Slow ☐ Average ☐ Rapid

Pain level: ☐ Mild ☐ Moderate ☐ Severe

Pain Location
(Mark with an "X")

Left, right, center: _____

Pain Description

☐ Throbbing   ☐ Piercing   ☐ Pounding

☐ Dull   ☐ Burning   ☐ Pulsating

☐ Constant   ☐ Debilitating   ☐ Squeezing

☐ Other _____

Symptoms

☐ Light sensitivity   ☐ Sound sensitivity   ☐ Aura   ☐ Confusion

☐ Dizziness   ☐ Nausea   ☐ Vomiting   ☐ Chills

☐ Muscle aches   ☐ Muscle stiffness   ☐ Restlessness   ☐ Congestion

☐ Coughing   ☐ Diarrhea   ☐ Fever   ☐ Sore throat

Other symptoms: _____

Health

Physical activity (past week):   ☐ Low   ☐ Moderate   ☐ High

Sleep quality (past week):   ☐ Poor   ☐ Average   ☐ Good

Computer time (past week):   ☐ Low   ☐ Moderate   ☐ High

Stress level (past 3 days):   ☐ Low   ☐ Moderate   ☐ High

Hormones

☐ PMS   ☐ Menstruation   ☐ Menopause   ☐ Puberty   ☐ Other: _____

Treatments Applied

Medication(s)/ dosage: _____

☐ Massage   ☐ Stretching/ yoga   ☐ Nerve stimulation device

☐ Heat/bath   ☐ Acupuncture   ☐ Ice packs

Other: _____

Weather/ Altitude

Temperature: Humidity: Barometric pressure:

Pollen level: ☐ Low   ☐ Moderate   ☐ High   Current elevation:

Food Tracking

	Today	Yesterday
Meals/ snacks:		

	Today	Yesterday
Vitamins/ supplements:		

	Today	Past 5 days
Alcoholic beverages:		
Caffeinated beverages:		
8oz glasses of water:		

Additional Notes

_____
_____
_____
_____
_____

Doctor's Notes

Dr. Name: _____ Specialty: _____ Date: _____

_____
_____
_____
_____
_____
_____

Entry #: _____ Date: _____ Duration: _____

Onset: ☐ Slow ☐ Average ☐ Rapid

Pain level: ☐ Mild ☐ Moderate ☐ Severe

Pain Location
(Mark with an "X")

Pain Description

☐ Throbbing ☐ Piercing ☐ Pounding

☐ Dull ☐ Burning ☐ Pulsating

☐ Constant ☐ Debilitating ☐ Squeezing

☐ Other _____

Left, right, center: _____

Symptoms

☐ Light sensitivity ☐ Sound sensitivity ☐ Aura ☐ Confusion

☐ Dizziness ☐ Nausea ☐ Vomiting ☐ Chills

☐ Muscle aches ☐ Muscle stiffness ☐ Restlessness ☐ Congestion

☐ Coughing ☐ Diarrhea ☐ Fever ☐ Sore throat

Other symptoms: _____

Health

Physical activity (past week): ☐ Low ☐ Moderate ☐ High

Sleep quality (past week): ☐ Poor ☐ Average ☐ Good

Computer time (past week): ☐ Low ☐ Moderate ☐ High

Stress level (past 3 days): ☐ Low ☐ Moderate ☐ High

Hormones

☐ PMS ☐ Menstruation ☐ Menopause ☐ Puberty ☐ Other: _____

Treatments Applied

Medication(s)/ dosage: _____

☐ Massage ☐ Stretching/ yoga ☐ Nerve stimulation device

☐ Heat/bath ☐ Acupuncture ☐ Ice packs

Other: _____

Weather/ Altitude

Temperature: _____ Humidity: _____ Barometric pressure: _____

Pollen level: ⬜ Low ⬜ Moderate ⬜ High Current elevation: _____

Food Tracking

	Today	Yesterday
Meals/ snacks:		

	Today	Yesterday
Vitamins/ supplements:		

	Today	Past 5 days
Alcoholic beverages:		
Caffeinated beverages:		
8oz glasses of water:		

Additional Notes

_____
_____
_____
_____
_____

Doctor's Notes

Dr. Name: _____ Specialty: _____ Date: _____

_____
_____
_____
_____
_____
_____

Entry #: _____ Date: _____ Duration: _____

Onset: ☐ Slow ☐ Average ☐ Rapid

Pain level: ☐ Mild ☐ Moderate ☐ Severe

Pain Location
(Mark with an "X")

Pain Description

☐ Throbbing ☐ Piercing ☐ Pounding

☐ Dull ☐ Burning ☐ Pulsating

☐ Constant ☐ Debilitating ☐ Squeezing

☐ Other _____

Left, right, center: _____

Symptoms

☐ Light sensitivity ☐ Sound sensitivity ☐ Aura ☐ Confusion

☐ Dizziness ☐ Nausea ☐ Vomiting ☐ Chills

☐ Muscle aches ☐ Muscle stiffness ☐ Restlessness ☐ Congestion

☐ Coughing ☐ Diarrhea ☐ Fever ☐ Sore throat

Other symptoms: _____

Health

Physical activity (past week): ☐ Low ☐ Moderate ☐ High

Sleep quality (past week): ☐ Poor ☐ Average ☐ Good

Computer time (past week): ☐ Low ☐ Moderate ☐ High

Stress level (past 3 days): ☐ Low ☐ Moderate ☐ High

Hormones

☐ PMS ☐ Menstruation ☐ Menopause ☐ Puberty ☐ Other:

Treatments Applied

Medication(s)/ dosage: _____

☐ Massage ☐ Stretching/ yoga ☐ Nerve stimulation device

☐ Heat/bath ☐ Acupuncture ☐ Ice packs

Other: _____

Weather/ Altitude

Temperature: _____ Humidity: _____ Barometric pressure: _____

Pollen level: ☐ Low   ☐ Moderate   ☐ High   Current elevation: _____

Food Tracking

	Today	Yesterday
Meals/ snacks:		

	Today	Yesterday
Vitamins/ supplements:		

	Today	Past 5 days
Alcoholic beverages:		
Caffeinated beverages:		
8oz glasses of water:		

Additional Notes

_____
_____
_____
_____
_____

Doctor's Notes

Dr. Name: _____ Specialty: _____ Date: _____

_____
_____
_____
_____
_____
_____

Entry #: _____ Date: _____ Duration: _____

Onset: ☐ Slow ☐ Average ☐ Rapid

Pain level: ☐ Mild ☐ Moderate ☐ Severe

Pain Location
(Mark with an "X")

Pain Description

☐ Throbbing ☐ Piercing ☐ Pounding

☐ Dull ☐ Burning ☐ Pulsating

☐ Constant ☐ Debilitating ☐ Squeezing

☐ Other _____

Left, right, center: _____

Symptoms

☐ Light sensitivity ☐ Sound sensitivity ☐ Aura ☐ Confusion

☐ Dizziness ☐ Nausea ☐ Vomiting ☐ Chills

☐ Muscle aches ☐ Muscle stiffness ☐ Restlessness ☐ Congestion

☐ Coughing ☐ Diarrhea ☐ Fever ☐ Sore throat

Other symptoms: _____

Health

Physical activity (past week): ☐ Low ☐ Moderate ☐ High

Sleep quality (past week): ☐ Poor ☐ Average ☐ Good

Computer time (past week): ☐ Low ☐ Moderate ☐ High

Stress level (past 3 days): ☐ Low ☐ Moderate ☐ High

Hormones

☐ PMS ☐ Menstruation ☐ Menopause ☐ Puberty ☐ Other: _____

Treatments Applied

Medication(s)/
dosage: _____

☐ Massage ☐ Stretching/ yoga ☐ Nerve stimulation device

☐ Heat/bath ☐ Acupuncture ☐ Ice packs

Other: _____

Weather/ Altitude

Temperature: Humidity: Barometric pressure:

Pollen level: ☐ Low   ☐ Moderate   ☐ High   Current elevation:

Food Tracking

	Today	Yesterday
Meals/ snacks:		

	Today	Yesterday
Vitamins/ supplements:		

	Today	Past 5 days
Alcoholic beverages:		
Caffeinated beverages:		
8oz glasses of water:		

Additional Notes

_____

_____

_____

_____

_____

Doctor's Notes

Dr. Name: _____ Specialty: _____ Date: _____

_____

_____

_____

_____

_____

_____

Entry #: _____ Date: _____ Duration: _____

Onset: ☐ Slow ☐ Average ☐ Rapid

Pain level: ☐ Mild ☐ Moderate ☐ Severe

Pain Location
(Mark with an "X")

Left, right, center: _____

Pain Description

☐ Throbbing ☐ Piercing ☐ Pounding

☐ Dull ☐ Burning ☐ Pulsating

☐ Constant ☐ Debilitating ☐ Squeezing

☐ Other _____

Symptoms

☐ Light sensitivity ☐ Sound sensitivity ☐ Aura ☐ Confusion

☐ Dizziness ☐ Nausea ☐ Vomiting ☐ Chills

☐ Muscle aches ☐ Muscle stiffness ☐ Restlessness ☐ Congestion

☐ Coughing ☐ Diarrhea ☐ Fever ☐ Sore throat

Other symptoms: _____

Health

Physical activity (past week): ☐ Low ☐ Moderate ☐ High

Sleep quality (past week): ☐ Poor ☐ Average ☐ Good

Computer time (past week): ☐ Low ☐ Moderate ☐ High

Stress level (past 3 days): ☐ Low ☐ Moderate ☐ High

Hormones

☐ PMS ☐ Menstruation ☐ Menopause ☐ Puberty ☐ Other: _____

Treatments Applied

Medication(s)/ dosage: _____

☐ Massage ☐ Stretching/ yoga ☐ Nerve stimulation device

☐ Heat/bath ☐ Acupuncture ☐ Ice packs

Other: _____

Weather/ Altitude

Temperature: _____ Humidity: _____ Barometric pressure: _____

Pollen level: ◯ Low ◯ Moderate ◯ High Current elevation: _____

Food Tracking

	Today	Yesterday
Meals/ snacks:		

	Today	Yesterday
Vitamins/ supplements:		

	Today	Past 5 days
Alcoholic beverages:		
Caffeinated beverages:		
8oz glasses of water:		

Additional Notes

_____
_____
_____
_____
_____

Doctor's Notes

Dr. Name: _____ Specialty: _____ Date: _____

_____
_____
_____
_____
_____
_____

Entry #: _____ Date: _____ Duration: _____

Onset: ☐ Slow ☐ Average ☐ Rapid

Pain level: ☐ Mild ☐ Moderate ☐ Severe

Pain Location
(Mark with an "X")

Pain Description

☐ Throbbing ☐ Piercing ☐ Pounding

☐ Dull ☐ Burning ☐ Pulsating

☐ Constant ☐ Debilitating ☐ Squeezing

☐ Other _____

Left, right, center: _____

Symptoms

☐ Light sensitivity ☐ Sound sensitivity ☐ Aura ☐ Confusion

☐ Dizziness ☐ Nausea ☐ Vomiting ☐ Chills

☐ Muscle aches ☐ Muscle stiffness ☐ Restlessness ☐ Congestion

☐ Coughing ☐ Diarrhea ☐ Fever ☐ Sore throat

Other symptoms: _____

Health

Physical activity (past week): ☐ Low ☐ Moderate ☐ High

Sleep quality (past week): ☐ Poor ☐ Average ☐ Good

Computer time (past week): ☐ Low ☐ Moderate ☐ High

Stress level (past 3 days): ☐ Low ☐ Moderate ☐ High

Hormones

☐ PMS ☐ Menstruation ☐ Menopause ☐ Puberty ☐ Other: _____

Treatments Applied

Medication(s)/
dosage: _____

☐ Massage ☐ Stretching/ yoga ☐ Nerve stimulation device

☐ Heat/bath ☐ Acupuncture ☐ Ice packs

Other: _____

Weather/ Altitude

Temperature: _____   Humidity: _____   Barometric pressure: _____

Pollen level: ☐ Low   ☐ Moderate   ☐ High   Current elevation: _____

Food Tracking

	Today	Yesterday
Meals/ snacks:		

	Today	Yesterday
Vitamins/ supplements:		

	Today	Past 5 days
Alcoholic beverages:		
Caffeinated beverages:		
8oz glasses of water:		

Additional Notes

_____
_____
_____
_____
_____

Doctor's Notes

Dr. Name: _____ Specialty: _____ Date: _____

_____
_____
_____
_____
_____
_____

Entry #: _____ Date: _____ Duration: _____

Onset: ☐ Slow ☐ Average ☐ Rapid

Pain level: ☐ Mild ☐ Moderate ☐ Severe

Pain Location
(Mark with an "X")

Pain Description

☐ Throbbing ☐ Piercing ☐ Pounding

☐ Dull ☐ Burning ☐ Pulsating

☐ Constant ☐ Debilitating ☐ Squeezing

☐ Other _____

Left, right, center: _____

Symptoms

☐ Light sensitivity ☐ Sound sensitivity ☐ Aura ☐ Confusion

☐ Dizziness ☐ Nausea ☐ Vomiting ☐ Chills

☐ Muscle aches ☐ Muscle stiffness ☐ Restlessness ☐ Congestion

☐ Coughing ☐ Diarrhea ☐ Fever ☐ Sore throat

Other symptoms: _____

Health

Physical activity (past week): ☐ Low ☐ Moderate ☐ High

Sleep quality (past week): ☐ Poor ☐ Average ☐ Good

Computer time (past week): ☐ Low ☐ Moderate ☐ High

Stress level (past 3 days): ☐ Low ☐ Moderate ☐ High

Hormones

☐ PMS ☐ Menstruation ☐ Menopause ☐ Puberty ☐ Other: _____

Treatments Applied

Medication(s)/ dosage: _____

☐ Massage ☐ Stretching/ yoga ☐ Nerve stimulation device

☐ Heat/bath ☐ Acupuncture ☐ Ice packs

Other: _____

Weather/ Altitude

Temperature: Humidity: Barometric pressure:

Pollen level: ☐ Low   ☐ Moderate   ☐ High   Current elevation:

Food Tracking

	Today	Yesterday
Meals/ snacks:		

	Today	Yesterday
Vitamins/ supplements:		

	Today	Past 5 days
Alcoholic beverages:		
Caffeinated beverages:		
8oz glasses of water:		

Additional Notes

_____
_____
_____
_____
_____

Doctor's Notes

Dr. Name: _____ Specialty: _____ Date: _____

_____
_____
_____
_____
_____
_____

Entry #: _____ Date: _____ Duration: _____

Onset: ☐ Slow ☐ Average ☐ Rapid

Pain level: ☐ Mild ☐ Moderate ☐ Severe

Pain Location
(Mark with an "X")

Pain Description

☐ Throbbing ☐ Piercing ☐ Pounding

☐ Dull ☐ Burning ☐ Pulsating

☐ Constant ☐ Debilitating ☐ Squeezing

☐ Other _____

Left, right, center: _____

Symptoms

☐ Light sensitivity ☐ Sound sensitivity ☐ Aura ☐ Confusion

☐ Dizziness ☐ Nausea ☐ Vomiting ☐ Chills

☐ Muscle aches ☐ Muscle stiffness ☐ Restlessness ☐ Congestion

☐ Coughing ☐ Diarrhea ☐ Fever ☐ Sore throat

Other symptoms: _____

Health

Physical activity (past week): ☐ Low ☐ Moderate ☐ High

Sleep quality (past week): ☐ Poor ☐ Average ☐ Good

Computer time (past week): ☐ Low ☐ Moderate ☐ High

Stress level (past 3 days): ☐ Low ☐ Moderate ☐ High

Hormones

☐ PMS ☐ Menstruation ☐ Menopause ☐ Puberty ☐ Other: _____

Treatments Applied

Medication(s)/ dosage: _____

☐ Massage ☐ Stretching/ yoga ☐ Nerve stimulation device

☐ Heat/bath ☐ Acupuncture ☐ Ice packs

Other: _____

Weather/ Altitude

Temperature: _____ Humidity: _____ Barometric pressure: _____

Pollen level: ( ) Low ( ) Moderate ( ) High Current elevation: _____

Food Tracking

	Today	Yesterday
Meals/ snacks:		

	Today	Yesterday
Vitamins/ supplements:		

	Today	Past 5 days
Alcoholic beverages:		
Caffeinated beverages:		
8oz glasses of water:		

Additional Notes

_____
_____
_____
_____
_____

Doctor's Notes

Dr. Name: _____ Specialty: _____ Date: _____

_____
_____
_____
_____
_____
_____

Entry #: _____ Date: _____ Duration: _____

Onset: ☐ Slow ☐ Average ☐ Rapid

Pain level: ☐ Mild ☐ Moderate ☐ Severe

Pain Location
(Mark with an "X")

Pain Description

☐ Throbbing ☐ Piercing ☐ Pounding

☐ Dull ☐ Burning ☐ Pulsating

☐ Constant ☐ Debilitating ☐ Squeezing

☐ Other _____

Left, right, center: _____

Symptoms

☐ Light sensitivity ☐ Sound sensitivity ☐ Aura ☐ Confusion

☐ Dizziness ☐ Nausea ☐ Vomiting ☐ Chills

☐ Muscle aches ☐ Muscle stiffness ☐ Restlessness ☐ Congestion

☐ Coughing ☐ Diarrhea ☐ Fever ☐ Sore throat

Other symptoms: _____

Health

Physical activity (past week): ☐ Low ☐ Moderate ☐ High

Sleep quality (past week): ☐ Poor ☐ Average ☐ Good

Computer time (past week): ☐ Low ☐ Moderate ☐ High

Stress level (past 3 days): ☐ Low ☐ Moderate ☐ High

Hormones

☐ PMS ☐ Menstruation ☐ Menopause ☐ Puberty ☐ Other: _____

Treatments Applied

Medication(s)/ dosage: _____

☐ Massage ☐ Stretching/ yoga ☐ Nerve stimulation device

☐ Heat/bath ☐ Acupuncture ☐ Ice packs

Other: _____

Weather/ Altitude

Temperature: Humidity: Barometric pressure:

Pollen level: ☐ Low   ☐ Moderate   ☐ High   Current elevation:

Food Tracking

	Today	Yesterday
Meals/ snacks:		

	Today	Yesterday
Vitamins/ supplements:		

	Today	Past 5 days
Alcoholic beverages:		
Caffeinated beverages:		
8oz glasses of water:		

Additional Notes

_____

_____

_____

_____

_____

Doctor's Notes

Dr. Name: _____ Specialty: _____ Date: _____

_____

_____

_____

_____

_____

_____

Entry #: _____ Date: _____ Duration: _____

Onset: ☐ Slow ☐ Average ☐ Rapid

Pain level: ☐ Mild ☐ Moderate ☐ Severe

Pain Location
(Mark with an "X")

Pain Description

☐ Throbbing ☐ Piercing ☐ Pounding

☐ Dull ☐ Burning ☐ Pulsating

☐ Constant ☐ Debilitating ☐ Squeezing

☐ Other _____

Left, right, center: _____

Symptoms

☐ Light sensitivity ☐ Sound sensitivity ☐ Aura ☐ Confusion

☐ Dizziness ☐ Nausea ☐ Vomiting ☐ Chills

☐ Muscle aches ☐ Muscle stiffness ☐ Restlessness ☐ Congestion

☐ Coughing ☐ Diarrhea ☐ Fever ☐ Sore throat

Other symptoms: _____

Health

Physical activity (past week): ☐ Low ☐ Moderate ☐ High

Sleep quality (past week): ☐ Poor ☐ Average ☐ Good

Computer time (past week): ☐ Low ☐ Moderate ☐ High

Stress level (past 3 days): ☐ Low ☐ Moderate ☐ High

Hormones

☐ PMS ☐ Menstruation ☐ Menopause ☐ Puberty ☐ Other: _____

Treatments Applied

Medication(s)/
dosage: _____

☐ Massage ☐ Stretching/ yoga ☐ Nerve stimulation device

☐ Heat/bath ☐ Acupuncture ☐ Ice packs

Other: _____

Weather/ Altitude

Temperature: Humidity: Barometric pressure:

Pollen level: ☐ Low ☐ Moderate ☐ High   Current elevation:

Food Tracking

	Today	Yesterday
Meals/ snacks:		

	Today	Yesterday
Vitamins/ supplements:		

	Today	Past 5 days
Alcoholic beverages:		
Caffeinated beverages:		
8oz glasses of water:		

Additional Notes

_____
_____
_____
_____
_____

Doctor's Notes

Dr. Name: _____ Specialty: _____ Date: _____

_____
_____
_____
_____
_____
_____

Entry #: _____ Date: _____ Duration: _____

Onset: ☐ Slow ☐ Average ☐ Rapid

Pain level: ☐ Mild ☐ Moderate ☐ Severe

Pain Location
(Mark with an "X")

Left, right, center: _____

Pain Description

☐ Throbbing ☐ Piercing ☐ Pounding

☐ Dull ☐ Burning ☐ Pulsating

☐ Constant ☐ Debilitating ☐ Squeezing

☐ Other _____

Symptoms

☐ Light sensitivity ☐ Sound sensitivity ☐ Aura ☐ Confusion

☐ Dizziness ☐ Nausea ☐ Vomiting ☐ Chills

☐ Muscle aches ☐ Muscle stiffness ☐ Restlessness ☐ Congestion

☐ Coughing ☐ Diarrhea ☐ Fever ☐ Sore throat

Other symptoms: _____

Health

Physical activity (past week): ☐ Low ☐ Moderate ☐ High

Sleep quality (past week): ☐ Poor ☐ Average ☐ Good

Computer time (past week): ☐ Low ☐ Moderate ☐ High

Stress level (past 3 days): ☐ Low ☐ Moderate ☐ High

Hormones

☐ PMS ☐ Menstruation ☐ Menopause ☐ Puberty ☐ Other: _____

Treatments Applied

Medication(s)/ dosage: _____

☐ Massage ☐ Stretching/ yoga ☐ Nerve stimulation device

☐ Heat/bath ☐ Acupuncture ☐ Ice packs

Other: _____

Weather/ Altitude

Temperature: _____ Humidity: _____ Barometric pressure: _____

Pollen level: ☐ Low ☐ Moderate ☐ High Current elevation: _____

Food Tracking

	Today	Yesterday
Meals/ snacks:		

	Today	Yesterday
Vitamins/ supplements:		

	Today	Past 5 days
Alcoholic beverages:		
Caffeinated beverages:		
8oz glasses of water:		

Additional Notes

_____
_____
_____
_____
_____

Doctor's Notes

Dr. Name: _____ Specialty: _____ Date: _____

_____
_____
_____
_____
_____
_____

Entry #: _____ Date: _____ Duration: _____

Onset: ☐ Slow ☐ Average ☐ Rapid

Pain level: ☐ Mild ☐ Moderate ☐ Severe

Pain Location
(Mark with an "X")

Left, right, center: _____

Pain Description

☐ Throbbing ☐ Piercing ☐ Pounding

☐ Dull ☐ Burning ☐ Pulsating

☐ Constant ☐ Debilitating ☐ Squeezing

☐ Other _____

Symptoms

☐ Light sensitivity ☐ Sound sensitivity ☐ Aura ☐ Confusion

☐ Dizziness ☐ Nausea ☐ Vomiting ☐ Chills

☐ Muscle aches ☐ Muscle stiffness ☐ Restlessness ☐ Congestion

☐ Coughing ☐ Diarrhea ☐ Fever ☐ Sore throat

Other symptoms: _____

Health

Physical activity (past week): ☐ Low ☐ Moderate ☐ High

Sleep quality (past week): ☐ Poor ☐ Average ☐ Good

Computer time (past week): ☐ Low ☐ Moderate ☐ High

Stress level (past 3 days): ☐ Low ☐ Moderate ☐ High

Hormones

☐ PMS ☐ Menstruation ☐ Menopause ☐ Puberty ☐ Other: _____

Treatments Applied

Medication(s)/ dosage: _____

☐ Massage ☐ Stretching/ yoga ☐ Nerve stimulation device

☐ Heat/bath ☐ Acupuncture ☐ Ice packs

Other: _____

Weather/ Altitude

Temperature: Humidity: Barometric pressure:

Pollen level: ☐ Low   ☐ Moderate   ☐ High   Current elevation:

Food Tracking

	Today	Yesterday
Meals/ snacks:		

	Today	Yesterday
Vitamins/ supplements:		

	Today	Past 5 days
Alcoholic beverages:		
Caffeinated beverages:		
8oz glasses of water:		

Additional Notes

_____
_____
_____
_____
_____

Doctor's Notes

Dr. Name: _____ Specialty: _____ Date: _____

_____
_____
_____
_____
_____
_____

Entry #: _____ Date: _____ Duration: _____

Onset: ☐ Slow ☐ Average ☐ Rapid

Pain level: ☐ Mild ☐ Moderate ☐ Severe

Pain Location
(Mark with an "X)

Pain Description

☐ Throbbing ☐ Piercing ☐ Pounding

☐ Dull ☐ Burning ☐ Pulsating

☐ Constant ☐ Debilitating ☐ Squeezing

☐ Other

Left, right, center:

Symptoms

☐ Light sensitivity ☐ Sound sensitivity ☐ Aura ☐ Confusion

☐ Dizziness ☐ Nausea ☐ Vomiting ☐ Chills

☐ Muscle aches ☐ Muscle stiffness ☐ Restlessness ☐ Congestion

☐ Coughing ☐ Diarrhea ☐ Fever ☐ Sore throat

Other symptoms:

Health

Physical activity (past week): ☐ Low ☐ Moderate ☐ High

Sleep quality (past week): ☐ Poor ☐ Average ☐ Good

Computer time (past week): ☐ Low ☐ Moderate ☐ High

Stress level (past 3 days): ☐ Low ☐ Moderate ☐ High

Hormones

☐ PMS ☐ Menstruation ☐ Menopause ☐ Puberty ☐ Other:

Treatments Applied

Medication(s)/
dosage:

☐ Massage ☐ Stretching/ yoga ☐ Nerve stimulation device

☐ Heat/bath ☐ Acupuncture ☐ Ice packs

Other:

Weather/ Altitude

Temperature: Humidity: Barometric pressure:

Pollen level: ☐ Low   ☐ Moderate   ☐ High   Current elevation:

Food Tracking

	Today	Yesterday
Meals/ snacks:		

	Today	Yesterday
Vitamins/ supplements:		

	Today	Past 5 days
Alcoholic beverages:		
Caffeinated beverages:		
8oz glasses of water:		

Additional Notes

_____
_____
_____
_____
_____

Doctor's Notes

Dr. Name: _____ Specialty: _____ Date: _____

_____
_____
_____
_____
_____
_____

Entry #: _____ Date: _____ Duration: _____

Onset: ☐ Slow ☐ Average ☐ Rapid

Pain level: ☐ Mild ☐ Moderate ☐ Severe

Pain Location
(Mark with an "X")

Pain Description

☐ Throbbing ☐ Piercing ☐ Pounding

☐ Dull ☐ Burning ☐ Pulsating

☐ Constant ☐ Debilitating ☐ Squeezing

☐ Other _____

Left, right, center: _____

Symptoms

☐ Light sensitivity ☐ Sound sensitivity ☐ Aura ☐ Confusion

☐ Dizziness ☐ Nausea ☐ Vomiting ☐ Chills

☐ Muscle aches ☐ Muscle stiffness ☐ Restlessness ☐ Congestion

☐ Coughing ☐ Diarrhea ☐ Fever ☐ Sore throat

Other symptoms: _____

Health

Physical activity (past week): ☐ Low ☐ Moderate ☐ High

Sleep quality (past week): ☐ Poor ☐ Average ☐ Good

Computer time (past week): ☐ Low ☐ Moderate ☐ High

Stress level (past 3 days): ☐ Low ☐ Moderate ☐ High

Hormones

☐ PMS ☐ Menstruation ☐ Menopause ☐ Puberty ☐ Other: _____

Treatments Applied

Medication(s)/ dosage: _____

☐ Massage ☐ Stretching/ yoga ☐ Nerve stimulation device

☐ Heat/bath ☐ Acupuncture ☐ Ice packs

Other: _____

Weather/ Altitude

Temperature: Humidity: Barometric pressure:

Pollen level: ☐ Low   ☐ Moderate   ☐ High   Current elevation:

Food Tracking

	Today	Yesterday
Meals/ snacks:		

	Today	Yesterday
Vitamins/ supplements:		

	Today	Past 5 days
Alcoholic beverages:		
Caffeinated beverages:		
8oz glasses of water:		

Additional Notes

_____
_____
_____
_____
_____

Doctor's Notes

Dr. Name: _____ Specialty: _____ Date: _____

_____
_____
_____
_____
_____
_____

Entry #: _____ Date: _____ Duration: _____

Onset: ☐ Slow ☐ Average ☐ Rapid

Pain level: ☐ Mild ☐ Moderate ☐ Severe

Pain Location
(Mark with an "X")

Pain Description

☐ Throbbing ☐ Piercing ☐ Pounding

☐ Dull ☐ Burning ☐ Pulsating

☐ Constant ☐ Debilitating ☐ Squeezing

☐ Other

Left, right, center:

Symptoms

☐ Light sensitivity ☐ Sound sensitivity ☐ Aura ☐ Confusion

☐ Dizziness ☐ Nausea ☐ Vomiting ☐ Chills

☐ Muscle aches ☐ Muscle stiffness ☐ Restlessness ☐ Congestion

☐ Coughing ☐ Diarrhea ☐ Fever ☐ Sore throat

Other symptoms:

Health

Physical activity (past week): ☐ Low ☐ Moderate ☐ High

Sleep quality (past week): ☐ Poor ☐ Average ☐ Good

Computer time (past week): ☐ Low ☐ Moderate ☐ High

Stress level (past 3 days): ☐ Low ☐ Moderate ☐ High

Hormones

☐ PMS ☐ Menstruation ☐ Menopause ☐ Puberty ☐ Other:

Treatments Applied

Medication(s)/ dosage:

☐ Massage ☐ Stretching/ yoga ☐ Nerve stimulation device

☐ Heat/bath ☐ Acupuncture ☐ Ice packs

Other:

Weather/ Altitude

Temperature: _____   Humidity: _____   Barometric pressure:

Pollen level: ☐ Low   ☐ Moderate   ☐ High   Current elevation:

Food Tracking

	Today	Yesterday
Meals/ snacks:		

	Today	Yesterday
Vitamins/ supplements:		

	Today	Past 5 days
Alcoholic beverages:		
Caffeinated beverages:		
8oz glasses of water:		

Additional Notes

_____
_____
_____
_____
_____

Doctor's Notes

Dr. Name: _____   Specialty: _____   Date: _____

_____
_____
_____
_____
_____
_____

Entry #: _____ Date: _____ Duration: _____

Onset: ☐ Slow ☐ Average ☐ Rapid

Pain level: ☐ Mild ☐ Moderate ☐ Severe

Pain Location
(Mark with an "X")

Pain Description

☐ Throbbing ☐ Piercing ☐ Pounding

☐ Dull ☐ Burning ☐ Pulsating

☐ Constant ☐ Debilitating ☐ Squeezing

☐ Other _____

Left, right, center: _____

Symptoms

☐ Light sensitivity ☐ Sound sensitivity ☐ Aura ☐ Confusion

☐ Dizziness ☐ Nausea ☐ Vomiting ☐ Chills

☐ Muscle aches ☐ Muscle stiffness ☐ Restlessness ☐ Congestion

☐ Coughing ☐ Diarrhea ☐ Fever ☐ Sore throat

Other symptoms: _____

Health

Physical activity (past week): ☐ Low ☐ Moderate ☐ High

Sleep quality (past week): ☐ Poor ☐ Average ☐ Good

Computer time (past week): ☐ Low ☐ Moderate ☐ High

Stress level (past 3 days): ☐ Low ☐ Moderate ☐ High

Hormones

☐ PMS ☐ Menstruation ☐ Menopause ☐ Puberty ☐ Other:

Treatments Applied

Medication(s)/ dosage: _____

☐ Massage ☐ Stretching/ yoga ☐ Nerve stimulation device

☐ Heat/bath ☐ Acupuncture ☐ Ice packs

Other: _____

Weather/ Altitude

Temperature: Humidity: Barometric pressure:

Pollen level: ☐ Low   ☐ Moderate   ☐ High   Current elevation:

Food Tracking

	Today	Yesterday
Meals/ snacks:		

	Today	Yesterday
Vitamins/ supplements:		

	Today	Past 5 days
Alcoholic beverages:		
Caffeinated beverages:		
8oz glasses of water:		

Additional Notes

_____

_____

_____

_____

_____

Doctor's Notes

Dr. Name: _____ Specialty: _____ Date: _____

_____

_____

_____

_____

_____

_____

Entry #: _____ Date: _____ Duration: _____

Onset: ☐ Slow ☐ Average ☐ Rapid

Pain level: ☐ Mild ☐ Moderate ☐ Severe

Pain Location
(Mark with an "X")

Left, right, center: _____

Pain Description

☐ Throbbing ☐ Piercing ☐ Pounding

☐ Dull ☐ Burning ☐ Pulsating

☐ Constant ☐ Debilitating ☐ Squeezing

☐ Other _____

Symptoms

☐ Light sensitivity ☐ Sound sensitivity ☐ Aura ☐ Confusion

☐ Dizziness ☐ Nausea ☐ Vomiting ☐ Chills

☐ Muscle aches ☐ Muscle stiffness ☐ Restlessness ☐ Congestion

☐ Coughing ☐ Diarrhea ☐ Fever ☐ Sore throat

Other symptoms: _____

Health

Physical activity (past week): ☐ Low ☐ Moderate ☐ High

Sleep quality (past week): ☐ Poor ☐ Average ☐ Good

Computer time (past week): ☐ Low ☐ Moderate ☐ High

Stress level (past 3 days): ☐ Low ☐ Moderate ☐ High

Hormones

☐ PMS ☐ Menstruation ☐ Menopause ☐ Puberty ☐ Other: _____

Treatments Applied

Medication(s)/ dosage: _____

☐ Massage ☐ Stretching/ yoga ☐ Nerve stimulation device

☐ Heat/bath ☐ Acupuncture ☐ Ice packs

Other: _____

Weather/ Altitude

Temperature: Humidity: Barometric pressure:

Pollen level: ☐ Low   ☐ Moderate   ☐ High   Current elevation:

Food Tracking

	Today	Yesterday
Meals/ snacks:		

	Today	Yesterday
Vitamins/ supplements:		

	Today	Past 5 days
Alcoholic beverages:		
Caffeinated beverages:		
8oz glasses of water:		

Additional Notes

_____
_____
_____
_____
_____

Doctor's Notes

Dr. Name: _____ Specialty: _____ Date: _____

_____
_____
_____
_____
_____
_____

Entry #: _____ Date: _____ Duration: _____

Onset: ☐ Slow ☐ Average ☐ Rapid

Pain level: ☐ Mild ☐ Moderate ☐ Severe

Pain Location
(Mark with an "X")

Pain Description

☐ Throbbing ☐ Piercing ☐ Pounding

☐ Dull ☐ Burning ☐ Pulsating

☐ Constant ☐ Debilitating ☐ Squeezing

☐ Other _____

Left, right, center: _____

Symptoms

☐ Light sensitivity ☐ Sound sensitivity ☐ Aura ☐ Confusion

☐ Dizziness ☐ Nausea ☐ Vomiting ☐ Chills

☐ Muscle aches ☐ Muscle stiffness ☐ Restlessness ☐ Congestion

☐ Coughing ☐ Diarrhea ☐ Fever ☐ Sore throat

Other symptoms: _____

Health

Physical activity (past week): ☐ Low ☐ Moderate ☐ High

Sleep quality (past week): ☐ Poor ☐ Average ☐ Good

Computer time (past week): ☐ Low ☐ Moderate ☐ High

Stress level (past 3 days): ☐ Low ☐ Moderate ☐ High

Hormones

☐ PMS ☐ Menstruation ☐ Menopause ☐ Puberty ☐ Other: _____

Treatments Applied

Medication(s)/ dosage: _____

☐ Massage ☐ Stretching/ yoga ☐ Nerve stimulation device

☐ Heat/bath ☐ Acupuncture ☐ Ice packs

Other: _____

Weather/ Altitude

Temperature: _____   Humidity: _____   Barometric pressure: _____

Pollen level: ☐ Low   ☐ Moderate   ☐ High   Current elevation: _____

Food Tracking

	Today	Yesterday
Meals/ snacks:		

	Today	Yesterday
Vitamins/ supplements:		

	Today	Past 5 days
Alcoholic beverages:		
Caffeinated beverages:		
8oz glasses of water:		

Additional Notes

_____
_____
_____
_____
_____

Doctor's Notes

Dr. Name: _____   Specialty: _____   Date: _____

_____
_____
_____
_____
_____
_____

Entry #: _____ Date: _____ Duration: _____

Onset: ☐ Slow ☐ Average ☐ Rapid

Pain level: ☐ Mild ☐ Moderate ☐ Severe

Pain Location
(Mark with an "X")

Pain Description

☐ Throbbing ☐ Piercing ☐ Pounding

☐ Dull ☐ Burning ☐ Pulsating

☐ Constant ☐ Debilitating ☐ Squeezing

☐ Other _____

Left, right, center: _____

Symptoms

☐ Light sensitivity ☐ Sound sensitivity ☐ Aura ☐ Confusion

☐ Dizziness ☐ Nausea ☐ Vomiting ☐ Chills

☐ Muscle aches ☐ Muscle stiffness ☐ Restlessness ☐ Congestion

☐ Coughing ☐ Diarrhea ☐ Fever ☐ Sore throat

Other symptoms: _____

Health

Physical activity (past week): ☐ Low ☐ Moderate ☐ High

Sleep quality (past week): ☐ Poor ☐ Average ☐ Good

Computer time (past week): ☐ Low ☐ Moderate ☐ High

Stress level (past 3 days): ☐ Low ☐ Moderate ☐ High

Hormones

☐ PMS ☐ Menstruation ☐ Menopause ☐ Puberty ☐ Other: _____

Treatments Applied

Medication(s)/ dosage: _____

☐ Massage ☐ Stretching/ yoga ☐ Nerve stimulation device

☐ Heat/bath ☐ Acupuncture ☐ Ice packs

Other: _____

Weather/ Altitude

Temperature: Humidity: Barometric pressure:

Pollen level: ☐ Low   ☐ Moderate   ☐ High   Current elevation:

Food Tracking

	Today	Yesterday
Meals/ snacks:		

	Today	Yesterday
Vitamins/ supplements:		

	Today	Past 5 days
Alcoholic beverages:		
Caffeinated beverages:		
8oz glasses of water:		

Additional Notes

_____
_____
_____
_____
_____

Doctor's Notes

Dr. Name: _____ Specialty: _____ Date: _____

_____
_____
_____
_____
_____
_____

Entry #: _____ Date: _____ Duration: _____

Onset: ☐ Slow ☐ Average ☐ Rapid

Pain level: ☐ Mild ☐ Moderate ☐ Severe

Pain Location
(Mark with an "X")

Pain Description

☐ Throbbing ☐ Piercing ☐ Pounding

☐ Dull ☐ Burning ☐ Pulsating

☐ Constant ☐ Debilitating ☐ Squeezing

☐ Other _____

Left, right, center: _____

Symptoms

☐ Light sensitivity ☐ Sound sensitivity ☐ Aura ☐ Confusion

☐ Dizziness ☐ Nausea ☐ Vomiting ☐ Chills

☐ Muscle aches ☐ Muscle stiffness ☐ Restlessness ☐ Congestion

☐ Coughing ☐ Diarrhea ☐ Fever ☐ Sore throat

Other symptoms: _____

Health

Physical activity (past week): ☐ Low ☐ Moderate ☐ High

Sleep quality (past week): ☐ Poor ☐ Average ☐ Good

Computer time (past week): ☐ Low ☐ Moderate ☐ High

Stress level (past 3 days): ☐ Low ☐ Moderate ☐ High

Hormones

☐ PMS ☐ Menstruation ☐ Menopause ☐ Puberty ☐ Other: _____

Treatments Applied

Medication(s)/ dosage: _____

☐ Massage ☐ Stretching/ yoga ☐ Nerve stimulation device

☐ Heat/bath ☐ Acupuncture ☐ Ice packs

Other: _____

Weather/ Altitude

Temperature: _____   Humidity: _____   Barometric pressure: _____

Pollen level: ☐ Low   ☐ Moderate   ☐ High   Current elevation: _____

Food Tracking

	Today	Yesterday
Meals/ snacks:		

	Today	Yesterday
Vitamins/ supplements:		

	Today	Past 5 days
Alcoholic beverages:		
Caffeinated beverages:		
8oz glasses of water:		

Additional Notes

_____
_____
_____
_____
_____

Doctor's Notes

Dr. Name: _____ Specialty: _____ Date: _____

_____
_____
_____
_____
_____
_____

Entry #: _____ Date: _____ Duration: _____

Pain Location
(Mark with an "X")

Onset: ☐ Slow ☐ Average ☐ Rapid

Pain level: ☐ Mild ☐ Moderate ☐ Severe

Pain Description

☐ Throbbing ☐ Piercing ☐ Pounding

☐ Dull ☐ Burning ☐ Pulsating

☐ Constant ☐ Debilitating ☐ Squeezing

☐ Other

Left, right, center:

Symptoms

☐ Light sensitivity ☐ Sound sensitivity ☐ Aura ☐ Confusion

☐ Dizziness ☐ Nausea ☐ Vomiting ☐ Chills

☐ Muscle aches ☐ Muscle stiffness ☐ Restlessness ☐ Congestion

☐ Coughing ☐ Diarrhea ☐ Fever ☐ Sore throat

Other symptoms:

Health

Physical activity (past week): ☐ Low ☐ Moderate ☐ High

Sleep quality (past week): ☐ Poor ☐ Average ☐ Good

Computer time (past week): ☐ Low ☐ Moderate ☐ High

Stress level (past 3 days): ☐ Low ☐ Moderate ☐ High

Hormones

☐ PMS ☐ Menstruation ☐ Menopause ☐ Puberty ☐ Other:

Treatments Applied

Medication(s)/
dosage:

☐ Massage ☐ Stretching/ yoga ☐ Nerve stimulation device

☐ Heat/bath ☐ Acupuncture ☐ Ice packs

Other:

Weather/ Altitude

Temperature: _____ Humidity: _____ Barometric pressure: _____

Pollen level: ☐ Low ☐ Moderate ☐ High Current elevation: _____

Food Tracking

	Today	Yesterday
Meals/ snacks:		

	Today	Yesterday
Vitamins/ supplements:		

	Today	Past 5 days
Alcoholic beverages:		
Caffeinated beverages:		
8oz glasses of water:		

Additional Notes

_____
_____
_____
_____
_____

Doctor's Notes

Dr. Name: _____ Specialty: _____ Date: _____

_____
_____
_____
_____
_____
_____

Entry #: _____ Date: _____ Duration: _____

Onset: ☐ Slow ☐ Average ☐ Rapid

Pain level: ☐ Mild ☐ Moderate ☐ Severe

Pain Location
(Mark with an "X")

Pain Description

☐ Throbbing ☐ Piercing ☐ Pounding

☐ Dull ☐ Burning ☐ Pulsating

☐ Constant ☐ Debilitating ☐ Squeezing

☐ Other _____

Left, right, center: _____

Symptoms

☐ Light sensitivity ☐ Sound sensitivity ☐ Aura ☐ Confusion

☐ Dizziness ☐ Nausea ☐ Vomiting ☐ Chills

☐ Muscle aches ☐ Muscle stiffness ☐ Restlessness ☐ Congestion

☐ Coughing ☐ Diarrhea ☐ Fever ☐ Sore throat

Other symptoms: _____

Health

Physical activity (past week): ☐ Low ☐ Moderate ☐ High

Sleep quality (past week): ☐ Poor ☐ Average ☐ Good

Computer time (past week): ☐ Low ☐ Moderate ☐ High

Stress level (past 3 days): ☐ Low ☐ Moderate ☐ High

Hormones

☐ PMS ☐ Menstruation ☐ Menopause ☐ Puberty ☐ Other: _____

Treatments Applied

Medication(s)/ dosage: _____

☐ Massage ☐ Stretching/ yoga ☐ Nerve stimulation device

☐ Heat/bath ☐ Acupuncture ☐ Ice packs

Other: _____

Weather/ Altitude

Temperature: ⬚ Humidity: ⬚ Barometric pressure:

Pollen level: ⬚ Low ⬚ Moderate ⬚ High Current elevation:

Food Tracking

	Today	Yesterday
Meals/ snacks:		

	Today	Yesterday
Vitamins/ supplements:		

	Today	Past 5 days
Alcoholic beverages:		
Caffeinated beverages:		
8oz glasses of water:		

Additional Notes

_____
_____
_____
_____
_____

Doctor's Notes

Dr. Name: _____ Specialty: _____ Date: _____

_____
_____
_____
_____
_____
_____

Entry #: _____ Date: _____ Duration: _____

Onset: ☐ Slow ☐ Average ☐ Rapid

Pain level: ☐ Mild ☐ Moderate ☐ Severe

Pain Location
(Mark with an "X")

Pain Description

☐ Throbbing ☐ Piercing ☐ Pounding

☐ Dull ☐ Burning ☐ Pulsating

☐ Constant ☐ Debilitating ☐ Squeezing

☐ Other _____

Left, right, center: _____

Symptoms

☐ Light sensitivity ☐ Sound sensitivity ☐ Aura ☐ Confusion

☐ Dizziness ☐ Nausea ☐ Vomiting ☐ Chills

☐ Muscle aches ☐ Muscle stiffness ☐ Restlessness ☐ Congestion

☐ Coughing ☐ Diarrhea ☐ Fever ☐ Sore throat

Other symptoms: _____

Health

Physical activity (past week): ☐ Low ☐ Moderate ☐ High

Sleep quality (past week): ☐ Poor ☐ Average ☐ Good

Computer time (past week): ☐ Low ☐ Moderate ☐ High

Stress level (past 3 days): ☐ Low ☐ Moderate ☐ High

Hormones

☐ PMS ☐ Menstruation ☐ Menopause ☐ Puberty ☐ Other: _____

Treatments Applied

Medication(s)/ dosage: _____

☐ Massage ☐ Stretching/ yoga ☐ Nerve stimulation device

☐ Heat/bath ☐ Acupuncture ☐ Ice packs

Other: _____

Weather/ Altitude

Temperature: Humidity: Barometric pressure:

Pollen level: ☐ Low   ☐ Moderate   ☐ High   Current elevation:

Food Tracking

	Today	Yesterday
Meals/ snacks:		

	Today	Yesterday
Vitamins/ supplements:		

	Today	Past 5 days
Alcoholic beverages:		
Caffeinated beverages:		
8oz glasses of water:		

Additional Notes

_____
_____
_____
_____
_____

Doctor's Notes

Dr. Name: _____ Specialty: _____ Date: _____

_____
_____
_____
_____
_____
_____

Entry #: _____ Date: _____ Duration: _____

Pain Location
(Mark with an "X")

Onset: ☐ Slow ☐ Average ☐ Rapid

Pain level: ☐ Mild ☐ Moderate ☐ Severe

Pain Description

☐ Throbbing ☐ Piercing ☐ Pounding

☐ Dull ☐ Burning ☐ Pulsating

☐ Constant ☐ Debilitating ☐ Squeezing

☐ Other _____

Left, right, center: _____

Symptoms

☐ Light sensitivity ☐ Sound sensitivity ☐ Aura ☐ Confusion

☐ Dizziness ☐ Nausea ☐ Vomiting ☐ Chills

☐ Muscle aches ☐ Muscle stiffness ☐ Restlessness ☐ Congestion

☐ Coughing ☐ Diarrhea ☐ Fever ☐ Sore throat

Other symptoms: _____

Health

Physical activity (past week): ☐ Low ☐ Moderate ☐ High

Sleep quality (past week): ☐ Poor ☐ Average ☐ Good

Computer time (past week): ☐ Low ☐ Moderate ☐ High

Stress level (past 3 days): ☐ Low ☐ Moderate ☐ High

Hormones

☐ PMS ☐ Menstruation ☐ Menopause ☐ Puberty ☐ Other: _____

Treatments Applied

Medication(s)/ dosage: _____

☐ Massage ☐ Stretching/ yoga ☐ Nerve stimulation device

☐ Heat/bath ☐ Acupuncture ☐ Ice packs

Other: _____

Weather/ Altitude

Temperature: _____   Humidity: _____   Barometric pressure: _____

Pollen level: ☐ Low   ☐ Moderate   ☐ High   Current elevation: _____

Food Tracking

	Today	Yesterday
Meals/ snacks:		

	Today	Yesterday
Vitamins/ supplements:		

	Today	Past 5 days
Alcoholic beverages:		
Caffeinated beverages:		
8oz glasses of water:		

Additional Notes

_____
_____
_____
_____
_____

Doctor's Notes

Dr. Name: _____   Specialty: _____   Date: _____

_____
_____
_____
_____
_____
_____

Entry #: _____ Date: _____ Duration: _____

Onset: ☐ Slow ☐ Average ☐ Rapid

Pain level: ☐ Mild ☐ Moderate ☐ Severe

Pain Location
(Mark with an "X")

Pain Description

☐ Throbbing ☐ Piercing ☐ Pounding

☐ Dull ☐ Burning ☐ Pulsating

☐ Constant ☐ Debilitating ☐ Squeezing

☐ Other

Left, right, center:

Symptoms

☐ Light sensitivity ☐ Sound sensitivity ☐ Aura ☐ Confusion

☐ Dizziness ☐ Nausea ☐ Vomiting ☐ Chills

☐ Muscle aches ☐ Muscle stiffness ☐ Restlessness ☐ Congestion

☐ Coughing ☐ Diarrhea ☐ Fever ☐ Sore throat

Other symptoms:

Health

Physical activity (past week): ☐ Low ☐ Moderate ☐ High

Sleep quality (past week): ☐ Poor ☐ Average ☐ Good

Computer time (past week): ☐ Low ☐ Moderate ☐ High

Stress level (past 3 days): ☐ Low ☐ Moderate ☐ High

Hormones

☐ PMS ☐ Menstruation ☐ Menopause ☐ Puberty ☐ Other:

Treatments Applied

Medication(s)/
dosage:

☐ Massage ☐ Stretching/ yoga ☐ Nerve stimulation device

☐ Heat/bath ☐ Acupuncture ☐ Ice packs

Other:

Weather/ Altitude

Temperature: Humidity: Barometric pressure:

Pollen level: ☐ Low   ☐ Moderate   ☐ High   Current elevation:

Food Tracking

	Today	Yesterday
Meals/ snacks:		

	Today	Yesterday
Vitamins/ supplements:		

	Today	Past 5 days
Alcoholic beverages:		
Caffeinated beverages:		
8oz glasses of water:		

Additional Notes

_____
_____
_____
_____
_____

Doctor's Notes

Dr. Name: _____ Specialty: _____ Date: _____

_____
_____
_____
_____
_____
_____

Entry #: _____ Date: _____ Duration: _____

Onset: ☐ Slow ☐ Average ☐ Rapid

Pain level: ☐ Mild ☐ Moderate ☐ Severe

Pain Description

☐ Throbbing ☐ Piercing ☐ Pounding

☐ Dull ☐ Burning ☐ Pulsating

☐ Constant ☐ Debilitating ☐ Squeezing

☐ Other _____

Left, right, center: _____

Symptoms

☐ Light sensitivity ☐ Sound sensitivity ☐ Aura ☐ Confusion

☐ Dizziness ☐ Nausea ☐ Vomiting ☐ Chills

☐ Muscle aches ☐ Muscle stiffness ☐ Restlessness ☐ Congestion

☐ Coughing ☐ Diarrhea ☐ Fever ☐ Sore throat

Other symptoms: _____

Health

Physical activity (past week): ☐ Low ☐ Moderate ☐ High

Sleep quality (past week): ☐ Poor ☐ Average ☐ Good

Computer time (past week): ☐ Low ☐ Moderate ☐ High

Stress level (past 3 days): ☐ Low ☐ Moderate ☐ High

Hormones

☐ PMS ☐ Menstruation ☐ Menopause ☐ Puberty ☐ Other: _____

Treatments Applied

Medication(s)/dosage: _____

☐ Massage ☐ Stretching/ yoga ☐ Nerve stimulation device

☐ Heat/bath ☐ Acupuncture ☐ Ice packs

Other: _____

Weather/ Altitude

Temperature: _____   Humidity: _____   Barometric pressure: _____

Pollen level: ◯ Low   ◯ Moderate   ◯ High   Current elevation: _____

Food Tracking

	Today	Yesterday
Meals/ snacks:		

	Today	Yesterday
Vitamins/ supplements:		

	Today	Past 5 days
Alcoholic beverages:		
Caffeinated beverages:		
8oz glasses of water:		

Additional Notes

_____
_____
_____
_____
_____

Doctor's Notes

Dr. Name: _____ Specialty: _____ Date: _____

_____
_____
_____
_____
_____
_____

Entry #: _____ Date: _____ Duration: _____

Onset: ☐ Slow ☐ Average ☐ Rapid

Pain level: ☐ Mild ☐ Moderate ☐ Severe

Pain Location
(Mark with an "X")

Pain Description

☐ Throbbing ☐ Piercing ☐ Pounding

☐ Dull ☐ Burning ☐ Pulsating

☐ Constant ☐ Debilitating ☐ Squeezing

☐ Other _____

Left, right, center: _____

Symptoms

☐ Light sensitivity ☐ Sound sensitivity ☐ Aura ☐ Confusion

☐ Dizziness ☐ Nausea ☐ Vomiting ☐ Chills

☐ Muscle aches ☐ Muscle stiffness ☐ Restlessness ☐ Congestion

☐ Coughing ☐ Diarrhea ☐ Fever ☐ Sore throat

Other symptoms: _____

Health

Physical activity (past week): ☐ Low ☐ Moderate ☐ High

Sleep quality (past week): ☐ Poor ☐ Average ☐ Good

Computer time (past week): ☐ Low ☐ Moderate ☐ High

Stress level (past 3 days): ☐ Low ☐ Moderate ☐ High

Hormones

☐ PMS ☐ Menstruation ☐ Menopause ☐ Puberty ☐ Other: _____

Treatments Applied

Medication(s)/ dosage: _____

☐ Massage ☐ Stretching/ yoga ☐ Nerve stimulation device

☐ Heat/bath ☐ Acupuncture ☐ Ice packs

Other: _____

Weather/ Altitude

Temperature: Humidity: Barometric pressure:

Pollen level: ☐ Low   ☐ Moderate   ☐ High   Current elevation:

Food Tracking

	Today	Yesterday
Meals/ snacks:		

	Today	Yesterday
Vitamins/ supplements:		

	Today	Past 5 days
Alcoholic beverages:		
Caffeinated beverages:		
8oz glasses of water:		

Additional Notes

_____
_____
_____
_____
_____

Doctor's Notes

Dr. Name: _____ Specialty: _____ Date: _____

_____
_____
_____
_____
_____
_____

Entry #: _____ Date: _____ Duration: _____

Onset: ☐ Slow ☐ Average ☐ Rapid

Pain level: ☐ Mild ☐ Moderate ☐ Severe

Pain Location

(Mark with an "X")

Pain Description

☐ Throbbing ☐ Piercing ☐ Pounding

☐ Dull ☐ Burning ☐ Pulsating

☐ Constant ☐ Debilitating ☐ Squeezing

☐ Other

Left, right, center:

Symptoms

☐ Light sensitivity ☐ Sound sensitivity ☐ Aura ☐ Confusion

☐ Dizziness ☐ Nausea ☐ Vomiting ☐ Chills

☐ Muscle aches ☐ Muscle stiffness ☐ Restlessness ☐ Congestion

☐ Coughing ☐ Diarrhea ☐ Fever ☐ Sore throat

Other symptoms:

Health

Physical activity (past week): ☐ Low ☐ Moderate ☐ High

Sleep quality (past week): ☐ Poor ☐ Average ☐ Good

Computer time (past week): ☐ Low ☐ Moderate ☐ High

Stress level (past 3 days): ☐ Low ☐ Moderate ☐ High

Hormones

☐ PMS ☐ Menstruation ☐ Menopause ☐ Puberty ☐ Other:

Treatments Applied

Medication(s)/ dosage:

☐ Massage ☐ Stretching/ yoga ☐ Nerve stimulation device

☐ Heat/bath ☐ Acupuncture ☐ Ice packs

Other:

Weather/ Altitude

Temperature: Humidity: Barometric pressure:

Pollen level: ☐ Low   ☐ Moderate   ☐ High   Current elevation:

Food Tracking

	Today	Yesterday
Meals/ snacks:		

	Today	Yesterday
Vitamins/ supplements:		

	Today	Past 5 days
Alcoholic beverages:		
Caffeinated beverages:		
8oz glasses of water:		

Additional Notes

_____
_____
_____
_____
_____

Doctor's Notes

Dr. Name: _____ Specialty: _____ Date: _____

_____
_____
_____
_____
_____
_____

Entry #: _____ Date: _____ Duration: _____

Pain Location
(Mark with an "X")

Onset: ☐ Slow ☐ Average ☐ Rapid

Pain level: ☐ Mild ☐ Moderate ☐ Severe

Pain Description

☐ Throbbing ☐ Piercing ☐ Pounding

☐ Dull ☐ Burning ☐ Pulsating

☐ Constant ☐ Debilitating ☐ Squeezing

☐ Other _____

Left, right, center: _____

Symptoms

☐ Light sensitivity ☐ Sound sensitivity ☐ Aura ☐ Confusion

☐ Dizziness ☐ Nausea ☐ Vomiting ☐ Chills

☐ Muscle aches ☐ Muscle stiffness ☐ Restlessness ☐ Congestion

☐ Coughing ☐ Diarrhea ☐ Fever ☐ Sore throat

Other symptoms: _____

Health

Physical activity (past week): ☐ Low ☐ Moderate ☐ High

Sleep quality (past week): ☐ Poor ☐ Average ☐ Good

Computer time (past week): ☐ Low ☐ Moderate ☐ High

Stress level (past 3 days): ☐ Low ☐ Moderate ☐ High

Hormones

☐ PMS ☐ Menstruation ☐ Menopause ☐ Puberty ☐ Other: _____

Treatments Applied

Medication(s)/
dosage: _____

☐ Massage ☐ Stretching/ yoga ☐ Nerve stimulation device

☐ Heat/bath ☐ Acupuncture ☐ Ice packs

Other: _____

Weather/ Altitude

Temperature: Humidity: Barometric pressure:

Pollen level: ☐ Low   ☐ Moderate   ☐ High   Current elevation:

Food Tracking

	Today	Yesterday
Meals/ snacks:		

	Today	Yesterday
Vitamins/ supplements:		

	Today	Past 5 days
Alcoholic beverages:		
Caffeinated beverages:		
8oz glasses of water:		

Additional Notes

_____
_____
_____
_____
_____

Doctor's Notes

Dr. Name: _____ Specialty: _____ Date: _____

_____
_____
_____
_____
_____
_____

Entry #: _____ Date: _____ Duration: _____

Onset: ☐ Slow ☐ Average ☐ Rapid

Pain level: ☐ Mild ☐ Moderate ☐ Severe

Pain Location
(Mark with an "X")

Pain Description

☐ Throbbing ☐ Piercing ☐ Pounding

☐ Dull ☐ Burning ☐ Pulsating

☐ Constant ☐ Debilitating ☐ Squeezing

☐ Other _____

Left, right, center: _____

Symptoms

☐ Light sensitivity ☐ Sound sensitivity ☐ Aura ☐ Confusion

☐ Dizziness ☐ Nausea ☐ Vomiting ☐ Chills

☐ Muscle aches ☐ Muscle stiffness ☐ Restlessness ☐ Congestion

☐ Coughing ☐ Diarrhea ☐ Fever ☐ Sore throat

Other symptoms: _____

Health

Physical activity (past week): ☐ Low ☐ Moderate ☐ High

Sleep quality (past week): ☐ Poor ☐ Average ☐ Good

Computer time (past week): ☐ Low ☐ Moderate ☐ High

Stress level (past 3 days): ☐ Low ☐ Moderate ☐ High

Hormones

☐ PMS ☐ Menstruation ☐ Menopause ☐ Puberty ☐ Other: _____

Treatments Applied

Medication(s)/ dosage: _____

☐ Massage ☐ Stretching/ yoga ☐ Nerve stimulation device

☐ Heat/bath ☐ Acupuncture ☐ Ice packs

Other: _____

Weather/ Altitude

Temperature: _____ Humidity: _____ Barometric pressure: _____

Pollen level: ☐ Low ☐ Moderate ☐ High   Current elevation: _____

Food Tracking

	Today	Yesterday
Meals/ snacks:		

	Today	Yesterday
Vitamins/ supplements:		

	Today	Past 5 days
Alcoholic beverages:		
Caffeinated beverages:		
8oz glasses of water:		

Additional Notes

_____
_____
_____
_____
_____

Doctor's Notes

Dr. Name: _____ Specialty: _____ Date: _____

_____
_____
_____
_____
_____

Entry #: _____ Date: _____ Duration: _____

Onset: ☐ Slow ☐ Average ☐ Rapid

Pain level: ☐ Mild ☐ Moderate ☐ Severe

Pain Location
(Mark with an "X")

Left, right, center: _____

Pain Description

☐ Throbbing ☐ Piercing ☐ Pounding

☐ Dull ☐ Burning ☐ Pulsating

☐ Constant ☐ Debilitating ☐ Squeezing

☐ Other _____

Symptoms

☐ Light sensitivity ☐ Sound sensitivity ☐ Aura ☐ Confusion

☐ Dizziness ☐ Nausea ☐ Vomiting ☐ Chills

☐ Muscle aches ☐ Muscle stiffness ☐ Restlessness ☐ Congestion

☐ Coughing ☐ Diarrhea ☐ Fever ☐ Sore throat

Other symptoms: _____

Health

Physical activity (past week): ☐ Low ☐ Moderate ☐ High

Sleep quality (past week): ☐ Poor ☐ Average ☐ Good

Computer time (past week): ☐ Low ☐ Moderate ☐ High

Stress level (past 3 days): ☐ Low ☐ Moderate ☐ High

Hormones

☐ PMS ☐ Menstruation ☐ Menopause ☐ Puberty ☐ Other: _____

Treatments Applied

Medication(s)/ dosage: _____

☐ Massage ☐ Stretching/ yoga ☐ Nerve stimulation device

☐ Heat/bath ☐ Acupuncture ☐ Ice packs

Other: _____

Weather/ Altitude

Temperature: _____ Humidity: _____ Barometric pressure: _____

Pollen level: ☐ Low ☐ Moderate ☐ High Current elevation: _____

Food Tracking

	Today	Yesterday
Meals/ snacks:		

	Today	Yesterday
Vitamins/ supplements:		

	Today	Past 5 days
Alcoholic beverages:		
Caffeinated beverages:		
8oz glasses of water:		

Additional Notes

_____
_____
_____
_____
_____

Doctor's Notes

Dr. Name: _____ Specialty: _____ Date: _____

_____
_____
_____
_____
_____
_____

Entry #: _____ Date: _____ Duration: _____

Onset: ☐ Slow ☐ Average ☐ Rapid

Pain level: ☐ Mild ☐ Moderate ☐ Severe

Pain Location
(Mark with an "X")

Pain Description

☐ Throbbing ☐ Piercing ☐ Pounding

☐ Dull ☐ Burning ☐ Pulsating

☐ Constant ☐ Debilitating ☐ Squeezing

☐ Other _____

Left, right, center: _____

Symptoms

☐ Light sensitivity ☐ Sound sensitivity ☐ Aura ☐ Confusion

☐ Dizziness ☐ Nausea ☐ Vomiting ☐ Chills

☐ Muscle aches ☐ Muscle stiffness ☐ Restlessness ☐ Congestion

☐ Coughing ☐ Diarrhea ☐ Fever ☐ Sore throat

Other symptoms: _____

Health

Physical activity (past week): ☐ Low ☐ Moderate ☐ High

Sleep quality (past week): ☐ Poor ☐ Average ☐ Good

Computer time (past week): ☐ Low ☐ Moderate ☐ High

Stress level (past 3 days): ☐ Low ☐ Moderate ☐ High

Hormones

☐ PMS ☐ Menstruation ☐ Menopause ☐ Puberty ☐ Other: _____

Treatments Applied

Medication(s)/ dosage: _____

☐ Massage ☐ Stretching/ yoga ☐ Nerve stimulation device

☐ Heat/bath ☐ Acupuncture ☐ Ice packs

Other: _____

Weather/ Altitude

Temperature: _____ Humidity: _____ Barometric pressure: _____

Pollen level: ☐ Low ☐ Moderate ☐ High Current elevation: _____

Food Tracking

	Today	Yesterday
Meals/ snacks:		

	Today	Yesterday
Vitamins/ supplements:		

	Today	Past 5 days
Alcoholic beverages:		
Caffeinated beverages:		
8oz glasses of water:		

Additional Notes

_____

_____

_____

_____

_____

Doctor's Notes

Dr. Name: _____ Specialty: _____ Date: _____

_____

_____

_____

_____

_____

_____

Entry #: _____ Date: _____ Duration: _____

Onset: ☐ Slow ☐ Average ☐ Rapid

Pain level: ☐ Mild ☐ Moderate ☐ Severe

Pain Location
(Mark with an "X")

Left, right, center: _____

Pain Description

☐ Throbbing ☐ Piercing ☐ Pounding

☐ Dull ☐ Burning ☐ Pulsating

☐ Constant ☐ Debilitating ☐ Squeezing

☐ Other _____

Symptoms

☐ Light sensitivity ☐ Sound sensitivity ☐ Aura ☐ Confusion

☐ Dizziness ☐ Nausea ☐ Vomiting ☐ Chills

☐ Muscle aches ☐ Muscle stiffness ☐ Restlessness ☐ Congestion

☐ Coughing ☐ Diarrhea ☐ Fever ☐ Sore throat

Other symptoms: _____

Health

Physical activity (past week): ☐ Low ☐ Moderate ☐ High

Sleep quality (past week): ☐ Poor ☐ Average ☐ Good

Computer time (past week): ☐ Low ☐ Moderate ☐ High

Stress level (past 3 days): ☐ Low ☐ Moderate ☐ High

Hormones

☐ PMS ☐ Menstruation ☐ Menopause ☐ Puberty ☐ Other: _____

Treatments Applied

Medication(s)/ dosage: _____

☐ Massage ☐ Stretching/ yoga ☐ Nerve stimulation device

☐ Heat/bath ☐ Acupuncture ☐ Ice packs

Other: _____

Weather/ Altitude

Temperature: _____ Humidity: _____ Barometric pressure: _____

Pollen level: ☐ Low ☐ Moderate ☐ High Current elevation: _____

Food Tracking

	Today	Yesterday
Meals/ snacks:		

	Today	Yesterday
Vitamins/ supplements:		

	Today	Past 5 days
Alcoholic beverages:		
Caffeinated beverages:		
8oz glasses of water:		

Additional Notes

_____

_____

_____

_____

_____

Doctor's Notes

Dr. Name: _____ Specialty: _____ Date: _____

_____

_____

_____

_____

_____

_____

Entry #: _____ Date: _____ Duration: _____

Onset: ☐ Slow ☐ Average ☐ Rapid

Pain level: ☐ Mild ☐ Moderate ☐ Severe

Pain Location
(Mark with an "X")

Pain Description

☐ Throbbing ☐ Piercing ☐ Pounding

☐ Dull ☐ Burning ☐ Pulsating

☐ Constant ☐ Debilitating ☐ Squeezing

☐ Other

Left, right, center:

Symptoms

☐ Light sensitivity ☐ Sound sensitivity ☐ Aura ☐ Confusion

☐ Dizziness ☐ Nausea ☐ Vomiting ☐ Chills

☐ Muscle aches ☐ Muscle stiffness ☐ Restlessness ☐ Congestion

☐ Coughing ☐ Diarrhea ☐ Fever ☐ Sore throat

Other symptoms:

Health

Physical activity (past week): ☐ Low ☐ Moderate ☐ High

Sleep quality (past week): ☐ Poor ☐ Average ☐ Good

Computer time (past week): ☐ Low ☐ Moderate ☐ High

Stress level (past 3 days): ☐ Low ☐ Moderate ☐ High

Hormones

☐ PMS ☐ Menstruation ☐ Menopause ☐ Puberty ☐ Other:

Treatments Applied

Medication(s)/
dosage:

☐ Massage ☐ Stretching/ yoga ☐ Nerve stimulation device

☐ Heat/bath ☐ Acupuncture ☐ Ice packs

Other:

Weather/ Altitude

Temperature: Humidity: Barometric pressure:

Pollen level: ☐ Low   ☐ Moderate   ☐ High   Current elevation:

Food Tracking

	Today	Yesterday
Meals/ snacks:		

	Today	Yesterday
Vitamins/ supplements:		

	Today	Past 5 days
Alcoholic beverages:		
Caffeinated beverages:		
8oz glasses of water:		

Additional Notes

_____
_____
_____
_____
_____

Doctor's Notes

Dr. Name: _____ Specialty: _____ Date: _____

_____
_____
_____
_____
_____
_____

Entry #: _____ Date: _____ Duration: _____

Pain Location
(Mark with an "X")

Onset: ☐ Slow ☐ Average ☐ Rapid

Pain level: ☐ Mild ☐ Moderate ☐ Severe

Pain Description

☐ Throbbing ☐ Piercing ☐ Pounding

☐ Dull ☐ Burning ☐ Pulsating

☐ Constant ☐ Debilitating ☐ Squeezing

☐ Other _____

Left, right, center: _____

Symptoms

☐ Light sensitivity ☐ Sound sensitivity ☐ Aura ☐ Confusion

☐ Dizziness ☐ Nausea ☐ Vomiting ☐ Chills

☐ Muscle aches ☐ Muscle stiffness ☐ Restlessness ☐ Congestion

☐ Coughing ☐ Diarrhea ☐ Fever ☐ Sore throat

Other symptoms: _____

Health

Physical activity (past week): ☐ Low ☐ Moderate ☐ High

Sleep quality (past week): ☐ Poor ☐ Average ☐ Good

Computer time (past week): ☐ Low ☐ Moderate ☐ High

Stress level (past 3 days): ☐ Low ☐ Moderate ☐ High

Hormones

☐ PMS ☐ Menstruation ☐ Menopause ☐ Puberty ☐ Other: _____

Treatments Applied

Medication(s)/ dosage: _____

☐ Massage ☐ Stretching/ yoga ☐ Nerve stimulation device

☐ Heat/bath ☐ Acupuncture ☐ Ice packs

Other: _____

Weather/ Altitude

Temperature: _____ Humidity: _____ Barometric pressure: _____

Pollen level: ☐ Low ☐ Moderate ☐ High Current elevation: _____

Food Tracking

	Today	Yesterday
Meals/ snacks:		

	Today	Yesterday
Vitamins/ supplements:		

	Today	Past 5 days
Alcoholic beverages:		
Caffeinated beverages:		
8oz glasses of water:		

Additional Notes

_____
_____
_____
_____
_____

Doctor's Notes

Dr. Name: _____ Specialty: _____ Date: _____

_____
_____
_____
_____
_____
_____

Entry #: _____ Date: _____ Duration: _____

Onset: ☐ Slow ☐ Average ☐ Rapid

Pain level: ☐ Mild ☐ Moderate ☐ Severe

Pain Location
(Mark with an "X")

Pain Description

☐ Throbbing ☐ Piercing ☐ Pounding

☐ Dull ☐ Burning ☐ Pulsating

☐ Constant ☐ Debilitating ☐ Squeezing

☐ Other _____

Left, right, center: _____

Symptoms

☐ Light sensitivity ☐ Sound sensitivity ☐ Aura ☐ Confusion

☐ Dizziness ☐ Nausea ☐ Vomiting ☐ Chills

☐ Muscle aches ☐ Muscle stiffness ☐ Restlessness ☐ Congestion

☐ Coughing ☐ Diarrhea ☐ Fever ☐ Sore throat

Other symptoms: _____

Health

Physical activity (past week): ☐ Low ☐ Moderate ☐ High

Sleep quality (past week): ☐ Poor ☐ Average ☐ Good

Computer time (past week): ☐ Low ☐ Moderate ☐ High

Stress level (past 3 days): ☐ Low ☐ Moderate ☐ High

Hormones

☐ PMS ☐ Menstruation ☐ Menopause ☐ Puberty ☐ Other:

Treatments Applied

Medication(s)/ dosage: _____

☐ Massage ☐ Stretching/ yoga ☐ Nerve stimulation device

☐ Heat/bath ☐ Acupuncture ☐ Ice packs

Other: _____

Weather/ Altitude

Temperature: _____ Humidity: _____ Barometric pressure: _____

Pollen level: ☐ Low ☐ Moderate ☐ High Current elevation: _____

Food Tracking

	Today	Yesterday
Meals/ snacks:		

	Today	Yesterday
Vitamins/ supplements:		

	Today	Past 5 days
Alcoholic beverages:		
Caffeinated beverages:		
8oz glasses of water:		

Additional Notes

_____
_____
_____
_____
_____

Doctor's Notes

Dr. Name: _____ Specialty: _____ Date: _____

_____
_____
_____
_____
_____
_____

Entry #: _____ Date: _____ Duration: _____

Onset: ☐ Slow ☐ Average ☐ Rapid

Pain level: ☐ Mild ☐ Moderate ☐ Severe

Pain Location

(Mark with an "X")

Pain Description

☐ Throbbing ☐ Piercing ☐ Pounding

☐ Dull ☐ Burning ☐ Pulsating

☐ Constant ☐ Debilitating ☐ Squeezing

☐ Other _____

Left, right, center:

Symptoms

☐ Light sensitivity ☐ Sound sensitivity ☐ Aura ☐ Confusion

☐ Dizziness ☐ Nausea ☐ Vomiting ☐ Chills

☐ Muscle aches ☐ Muscle stiffness ☐ Restlessness ☐ Congestion

☐ Coughing ☐ Diarrhea ☐ Fever ☐ Sore throat

Other symptoms: _____

Health

Physical activity (past week): ☐ Low ☐ Moderate ☐ High

Sleep quality (past week): ☐ Poor ☐ Average ☐ Good

Computer time (past week): ☐ Low ☐ Moderate ☐ High

Stress level (past 3 days): ☐ Low ☐ Moderate ☐ High

Hormones

☐ PMS ☐ Menstruation ☐ Menopause ☐ Puberty ☐ Other: ____

Treatments Applied

Medication(s)/ dosage: _____

☐ Massage ☐ Stretching/ yoga ☐ Nerve stimulation device

☐ Heat/bath ☐ Acupuncture ☐ Ice packs

Other: _____

Weather/ Altitude

Temperature: Humidity: Barometric pressure:

Pollen level: ☐ Low   ☐ Moderate   ☐ High   Current elevation:

Food Tracking

	Today	Yesterday
Meals/ snacks:		

	Today	Yesterday
Vitamins/ supplements:		

	Today	Past 5 days
Alcoholic beverages:		
Caffeinated beverages:		
8oz glasses of water:		

Additional Notes

_____
_____
_____
_____
_____

Doctor's Notes

Dr. Name: _____ Specialty: _____ Date: _____

_____
_____
_____
_____
_____
_____

Entry #: _____ Date: _____ Duration: _____

Onset: ☐ Slow ☐ Average ☐ Rapid

Pain level: ☐ Mild ☐ Moderate ☐ Severe

Pain Location
(Mark with an "X")

Pain Description

☐ Throbbing ☐ Piercing ☐ Pounding

☐ Dull ☐ Burning ☐ Pulsating

☐ Constant ☐ Debilitating ☐ Squeezing

☐ Other _____

Left, right, center: _____

Symptoms

☐ Light sensitivity ☐ Sound sensitivity ☐ Aura ☐ Confusion

☐ Dizziness ☐ Nausea ☐ Vomiting ☐ Chills

☐ Muscle aches ☐ Muscle stiffness ☐ Restlessness ☐ Congestion

☐ Coughing ☐ Diarrhea ☐ Fever ☐ Sore throat

Other symptoms: _____

Health

Physical activity (past week): ☐ Low ☐ Moderate ☐ High

Sleep quality (past week): ☐ Poor ☐ Average ☐ Good

Computer time (past week): ☐ Low ☐ Moderate ☐ High

Stress level (past 3 days): ☐ Low ☐ Moderate ☐ High

Hormones

☐ PMS ☐ Menstruation ☐ Menopause ☐ Puberty ☐ Other: _____

Treatments Applied

Medication(s)/ dosage: _____

☐ Massage ☐ Stretching/ yoga ☐ Nerve stimulation device

☐ Heat/bath ☐ Acupuncture ☐ Ice packs

Other: _____

Weather/ Altitude

Temperature: [____]   Humidity: [____]   Barometric pressure: [____]

Pollen level: ◯ Low   ◯ Moderate   ◯ High   Current elevation: [____]

Food Tracking

	Today	Yesterday
Meals/ snacks:		

	Today	Yesterday
Vitamins/ supplements:		

	Today	Past 5 days
Alcoholic beverages:		
Caffeinated beverages:		
8oz glasses of water:		

Additional Notes

_____
_____
_____
_____
_____

Doctor's Notes

Dr. Name: _____ Specialty: _____ Date: _____

_____
_____
_____
_____
_____
_____

Entry #: _____ Date: _____ Duration: _____

Onset: ☐ Slow ☐ Average ☐ Rapid

Pain level: ☐ Mild ☐ Moderate ☐ Severe

Pain Location
(Mark with an "X")

Left, right, center: _____

Pain Description

☐ Throbbing ☐ Piercing ☐ Pounding

☐ Dull ☐ Burning ☐ Pulsating

☐ Constant ☐ Debilitating ☐ Squeezing

☐ Other _____

Symptoms

☐ Light sensitivity ☐ Sound sensitivity ☐ Aura ☐ Confusion

☐ Dizziness ☐ Nausea ☐ Vomiting ☐ Chills

☐ Muscle aches ☐ Muscle stiffness ☐ Restlessness ☐ Congestion

☐ Coughing ☐ Diarrhea ☐ Fever ☐ Sore throat

Other symptoms: _____

Health

Physical activity (past week): ☐ Low ☐ Moderate ☐ High

Sleep quality (past week): ☐ Poor ☐ Average ☐ Good

Computer time (past week): ☐ Low ☐ Moderate ☐ High

Stress level (past 3 days): ☐ Low ☐ Moderate ☐ High

Hormones

☐ PMS ☐ Menstruation ☐ Menopause ☐ Puberty ☐ Other: _____

Treatments Applied

Medication(s)/ dosage: _____

☐ Massage ☐ Stretching/ yoga ☐ Nerve stimulation device

☐ Heat/bath ☐ Acupuncture ☐ Ice packs

Other: _____

Weather/ Altitude

Temperature: _____   Humidity: _____   Barometric pressure: _____

Pollen level: ☐ Low   ☐ Moderate   ☐ High   Current elevation: _____

Food Tracking

	Today	Yesterday
Meals/ snacks:		

	Today	Yesterday
Vitamins/ supplements:		

	Today	Past 5 days
Alcoholic beverages:		
Caffeinated beverages:		
8oz glasses of water:		

Additional Notes

_____
_____
_____
_____
_____

Doctor's Notes

Dr. Name: _____ Specialty: _____ Date: _____

_____
_____
_____
_____
_____
_____

Entry #: _____ Date: _____ Duration: _____

Onset: ☐ Slow ☐ Average ☐ Rapid

Pain level: ☐ Mild ☐ Moderate ☐ Severe

Pain Location
(Mark with an "X")

Pain Description

☐ Throbbing ☐ Piercing ☐ Pounding

☐ Dull ☐ Burning ☐ Pulsating

☐ Constant ☐ Debilitating ☐ Squeezing

☐ Other _____

Left, right, center: _____

Symptoms

☐ Light sensitivity ☐ Sound sensitivity ☐ Aura ☐ Confusion

☐ Dizziness ☐ Nausea ☐ Vomiting ☐ Chills

☐ Muscle aches ☐ Muscle stiffness ☐ Restlessness ☐ Congestion

☐ Coughing ☐ Diarrhea ☐ Fever ☐ Sore throat

Other symptoms: _____

Health

Physical activity (past week): ☐ Low ☐ Moderate ☐ High

Sleep quality (past week): ☐ Poor ☐ Average ☐ Good

Computer time (past week): ☐ Low ☐ Moderate ☐ High

Stress level (past 3 days): ☐ Low ☐ Moderate ☐ High

Hormones

☐ PMS ☐ Menstruation ☐ Menopause ☐ Puberty ☐ Other: _____

Treatments Applied

Medication(s)/ dosage: _____

☐ Massage ☐ Stretching/ yoga ☐ Nerve stimulation device

☐ Heat/bath ☐ Acupuncture ☐ Ice packs

Other: _____

Weather/ Altitude

Temperature: Humidity: Barometric pressure:

Pollen level: ☐ Low ☐ Moderate ☐ High   Current elevation:

Food Tracking

	Today	Yesterday
Meals/ snacks:		

	Today	Yesterday
Vitamins/ supplements:		

	Today	Past 5 days
Alcoholic beverages:		
Caffeinated beverages:		
8oz glasses of water:		

Additional Notes

_____

_____

_____

_____

_____

Doctor's Notes

Dr. Name: _____ Specialty: _____ Date: _____

_____

_____

_____

_____

_____

_____

Entry #: _____ Date: _____ Duration: _____

Onset: ☐ Slow ☐ Average ☐ Rapid

Pain level: ☐ Mild ☐ Moderate ☐ Severe

Pain Location
(Mark with an "X")

Pain Description

☐ Throbbing ☐ Piercing ☐ Pounding

☐ Dull ☐ Burning ☐ Pulsating

☐ Constant ☐ Debilitating ☐ Squeezing

☐ Other _____

Left, right, center: _____

Symptoms

☐ Light sensitivity ☐ Sound sensitivity ☐ Aura ☐ Confusion

☐ Dizziness ☐ Nausea ☐ Vomiting ☐ Chills

☐ Muscle aches ☐ Muscle stiffness ☐ Restlessness ☐ Congestion

☐ Coughing ☐ Diarrhea ☐ Fever ☐ Sore throat

Other symptoms: _____

Health

Physical activity (past week): ☐ Low ☐ Moderate ☐ High

Sleep quality (past week): ☐ Poor ☐ Average ☐ Good

Computer time (past week): ☐ Low ☐ Moderate ☐ High

Stress level (past 3 days): ☐ Low ☐ Moderate ☐ High

Hormones

☐ PMS ☐ Menstruation ☐ Menopause ☐ Puberty ☐ Other: _____

Treatments Applied

Medication(s)/ dosage: _____

☐ Massage ☐ Stretching/ yoga ☐ Nerve stimulation device

☐ Heat/bath ☐ Acupuncture ☐ Ice packs

Other: _____

Weather/ Altitude

Temperature: _____ Humidity: _____ Barometric pressure: _____

Pollen level: ☐ Low ☐ Moderate ☐ High Current elevation: _____

Food Tracking

	Today	Yesterday
Meals/ snacks:		

	Today	Yesterday
Vitamins/ supplements:		

	Today	Past 5 days
Alcoholic beverages:		
Caffeinated beverages:		
8oz glasses of water:		

Additional Notes

_____
_____
_____
_____
_____

Doctor's Notes

Dr. Name: _____ Specialty: _____ Date: _____

_____
_____
_____
_____
_____
_____

Entry #: _____ Date: _____ Duration: _____

Onset: ☐ Slow ☐ Average ☐ Rapid

Pain level: ☐ Mild ☐ Moderate ☐ Severe

Pain Description

☐ Throbbing ☐ Piercing ☐ Pounding

☐ Dull ☐ Burning ☐ Pulsating

☐ Constant ☐ Debilitating ☐ Squeezing

☐ Other _____

Left, right, center: _____

Symptoms

☐ Light sensitivity ☐ Sound sensitivity ☐ Aura ☐ Confusion

☐ Dizziness ☐ Nausea ☐ Vomiting ☐ Chills

☐ Muscle aches ☐ Muscle stiffness ☐ Restlessness ☐ Congestion

☐ Coughing ☐ Diarrhea ☐ Fever ☐ Sore throat

Other symptoms: _____

Health

Physical activity (past week): ☐ Low ☐ Moderate ☐ High

Sleep quality (past week): ☐ Poor ☐ Average ☐ Good

Computer time (past week): ☐ Low ☐ Moderate ☐ High

Stress level (past 3 days): ☐ Low ☐ Moderate ☐ High

Hormones

☐ PMS ☐ Menstruation ☐ Menopause ☐ Puberty ☐ Other: _____

Treatments Applied

Medication(s)/ dosage: _____

☐ Massage ☐ Stretching/ yoga ☐ Nerve stimulation device

☐ Heat/bath ☐ Acupuncture ☐ Ice packs

Other: _____

Weather/ Altitude

Temperature: _____   Humidity: _____   Barometric pressure:

Pollen level: ☐ Low   ☐ Moderate   ☐ High   Current elevation:

Food Tracking

	Today	Yesterday
Meals/ snacks:		

	Today	Yesterday
Vitamins/ supplements:		

	Today	Past 5 days
Alcoholic beverages:		
Caffeinated beverages:		
8oz glasses of water:		

Additional Notes

_____
_____
_____
_____
_____

Doctor's Notes

Dr. Name: _____ Specialty: _____ Date: _____

_____
_____
_____
_____
_____
_____

Entry #: _____ Date: _____ Duration: _____

Onset: ☐ Slow ☐ Average ☐ Rapid

Pain level: ☐ Mild ☐ Moderate ☐ Severe

Pain Location
(Mark with an "X")

Left, right, center: _____

Pain Description

☐ Throbbing ☐ Piercing ☐ Pounding

☐ Dull ☐ Burning ☐ Pulsating

☐ Constant ☐ Debilitating ☐ Squeezing

☐ Other _____

Symptoms

☐ Light sensitivity ☐ Sound sensitivity ☐ Aura ☐ Confusion

☐ Dizziness ☐ Nausea ☐ Vomiting ☐ Chills

☐ Muscle aches ☐ Muscle stiffness ☐ Restlessness ☐ Congestion

☐ Coughing ☐ Diarrhea ☐ Fever ☐ Sore throat

Other symptoms: _____

Health

Physical activity (past week): ☐ Low ☐ Moderate ☐ High

Sleep quality (past week): ☐ Poor ☐ Average ☐ Good

Computer time (past week): ☐ Low ☐ Moderate ☐ High

Stress level (past 3 days): ☐ Low ☐ Moderate ☐ High

Hormones

☐ PMS ☐ Menstruation ☐ Menopause ☐ Puberty ☐ Other: _____

Treatments Applied

Medication(s)/ dosage: _____

☐ Massage ☐ Stretching/ yoga ☐ Nerve stimulation device

☐ Heat/bath ☐ Acupuncture ☐ Ice packs

Other: _____

Weather/ Altitude

Temperature: Humidity: Barometric pressure:

Pollen level: ☐ Low   ☐ Moderate   ☐ High   Current elevation:

Food Tracking

	Today	Yesterday
Meals/ snacks:		

	Today	Yesterday
Vitamins/ supplements:		

	Today	Past 5 days
Alcoholic beverages:		
Caffeinated beverages:		
8oz glasses of water:		

Additional Notes

_____
_____
_____
_____
_____

Doctor's Notes

Dr. Name: _____ Specialty: _____ Date: _____

_____
_____
_____
_____
_____
_____

Entry #: _____ Date: _____ Duration: _____

Onset: ☐ Slow ☐ Average ☐ Rapid

Pain level: ☐ Mild ☐ Moderate ☐ Severe

Pain Location
(Mark with an "X")

Pain Description

☐ Throbbing ☐ Piercing ☐ Pounding

☐ Dull ☐ Burning ☐ Pulsating

☐ Constant ☐ Debilitating ☐ Squeezing

☐ Other _____

Left, right, center: _____

Symptoms

☐ Light sensitivity ☐ Sound sensitivity ☐ Aura ☐ Confusion

☐ Dizziness ☐ Nausea ☐ Vomiting ☐ Chills

☐ Muscle aches ☐ Muscle stiffness ☐ Restlessness ☐ Congestion

☐ Coughing ☐ Diarrhea ☐ Fever ☐ Sore throat

Other symptoms: _____

Health

Physical activity (past week): ☐ Low ☐ Moderate ☐ High

Sleep quality (past week): ☐ Poor ☐ Average ☐ Good

Computer time (past week): ☐ Low ☐ Moderate ☐ High

Stress level (past 3 days): ☐ Low ☐ Moderate ☐ High

Hormones

☐ PMS ☐ Menstruation ☐ Menopause ☐ Puberty ☐ Other: _____

Treatments Applied

Medication(s)/ dosage: _____

☐ Massage ☐ Stretching/ yoga ☐ Nerve stimulation device

☐ Heat/bath ☐ Acupuncture ☐ Ice packs

Other: _____

Weather/ Altitude

Temperature: _____   Humidity: _____   Barometric pressure: _____

Pollen level: ☐ Low   ☐ Moderate   ☐ High   Current elevation: _____

Food Tracking

	Today	Yesterday
Meals/ snacks:		

	Today	Yesterday
Vitamins/ supplements:		

	Today	Past 5 days
Alcoholic beverages:		
Caffeinated beverages:		
8oz glasses of water:		

Additional Notes

_____
_____
_____
_____
_____

Doctor's Notes

Dr. Name: _____   Specialty: _____   Date: _____

_____
_____
_____
_____
_____
_____

Entry #: _____ Date: _____ Duration: _____

Onset: ☐ Slow ☐ Average ☐ Rapid

Pain level: ☐ Mild ☐ Moderate ☐ Severe

Pain Location
(Mark with an "X")

Pain Description

☐ Throbbing ☐ Piercing ☐ Pounding

☐ Dull ☐ Burning ☐ Pulsating

☐ Constant ☐ Debilitating ☐ Squeezing

☐ Other _____

Left, right, center: _____

Symptoms

☐ Light sensitivity ☐ Sound sensitivity ☐ Aura ☐ Confusion

☐ Dizziness ☐ Nausea ☐ Vomiting ☐ Chills

☐ Muscle aches ☐ Muscle stiffness ☐ Restlessness ☐ Congestion

☐ Coughing ☐ Diarrhea ☐ Fever ☐ Sore throat

Other symptoms: _____

Health

Physical activity (past week): ☐ Low ☐ Moderate ☐ High

Sleep quality (past week): ☐ Poor ☐ Average ☐ Good

Computer time (past week): ☐ Low ☐ Moderate ☐ High

Stress level (past 3 days): ☐ Low ☐ Moderate ☐ High

Hormones

☐ PMS ☐ Menstruation ☐ Menopause ☐ Puberty ☐ Other:

Treatments Applied

Medication(s)/ dosage: _____

☐ Massage ☐ Stretching/ yoga ☐ Nerve stimulation device

☐ Heat/bath ☐ Acupuncture ☐ Ice packs

Other: _____

Weather/ Altitude

Temperature: _____ Humidity: _____ Barometric pressure: _____

Pollen level: ☐ Low ☐ Moderate ☐ High Current elevation: _____

Food Tracking

	Today	Yesterday
Meals/ snacks:		

	Today	Yesterday
Vitamins/ supplements:		

	Today	Past 5 days
Alcoholic beverages:		
Caffeinated beverages:		
8oz glasses of water:		

Additional Notes

_____
_____
_____
_____
_____

Doctor's Notes

Dr. Name: _____ Specialty: _____ Date: _____

_____
_____
_____
_____
_____
_____

Entry #: _____ Date: _____ Duration: _____

Onset: ☐ Slow ☐ Average ☐ Rapid

Pain level: ☐ Mild ☐ Moderate ☐ Severe

Pain Location
(Mark with an "X)

Pain Description

☐ Throbbing ☐ Piercing ☐ Pounding

☐ Dull ☐ Burning ☐ Pulsating

☐ Constant ☐ Debilitating ☐ Squeezing

☐ Other _____

Left, right, center: _____

Symptoms

☐ Light sensitivity ☐ Sound sensitivity ☐ Aura ☐ Confusion

☐ Dizziness ☐ Nausea ☐ Vomiting ☐ Chills

☐ Muscle aches ☐ Muscle stiffness ☐ Restlessness ☐ Congestion

☐ Coughing ☐ Diarrhea ☐ Fever ☐ Sore throat

Other symptoms: _____

Health

Physical activity (past week): ☐ Low ☐ Moderate ☐ High

Sleep quality (past week): ☐ Poor ☐ Average ☐ Good

Computer time (past week): ☐ Low ☐ Moderate ☐ High

Stress level (past 3 days): ☐ Low ☐ Moderate ☐ High

Hormones

☐ PMS ☐ Menstruation ☐ Menopause ☐ Puberty ☐ Other: _____

Treatments Applied

Medication(s)/ dosage: _____

☐ Massage ☐ Stretching/ yoga ☐ Nerve stimulation device

☐ Heat/bath ☐ Acupuncture ☐ Ice packs

Other: _____

Weather/ Altitude

Temperature: Humidity: Barometric pressure:

Pollen level: ☐ Low   ☐ Moderate   ☐ High   Current elevation:

Food Tracking

	Today	Yesterday
Meals/ snacks:		

	Today	Yesterday
Vitamins/ supplements:		

	Today	Past 5 days
Alcoholic beverages:		
Caffeinated beverages:		
8oz glasses of water:		

Additional Notes

_____
_____
_____
_____
_____

Doctor's Notes

Dr. Name: _____ Specialty: _____ Date: _____

_____
_____
_____
_____
_____
_____

Entry #: _____ Date: _____ Duration: _____

Onset: ☐ Slow ☐ Average ☐ Rapid

Pain level: ☐ Mild ☐ Moderate ☐ Severe

Pain Location
(Mark with an "X")

Pain Description

☐ Throbbing ☐ Piercing ☐ Pounding

☐ Dull ☐ Burning ☐ Pulsating

☐ Constant ☐ Debilitating ☐ Squeezing

☐ Other _____

Left, right, center: _____

Symptoms

☐ Light sensitivity ☐ Sound sensitivity ☐ Aura ☐ Confusion

☐ Dizziness ☐ Nausea ☐ Vomiting ☐ Chills

☐ Muscle aches ☐ Muscle stiffness ☐ Restlessness ☐ Congestion

☐ Coughing ☐ Diarrhea ☐ Fever ☐ Sore throat

Other symptoms: _____

Health

Physical activity (past week): ☐ Low ☐ Moderate ☐ High

Sleep quality (past week): ☐ Poor ☐ Average ☐ Good

Computer time (past week): ☐ Low ☐ Moderate ☐ High

Stress level (past 3 days): ☐ Low ☐ Moderate ☐ High

Hormones

☐ PMS ☐ Menstruation ☐ Menopause ☐ Puberty ☐ Other: _____

Treatments Applied

Medication(s)/ dosage: _____

☐ Massage ☐ Stretching/ yoga ☐ Nerve stimulation device

☐ Heat/bath ☐ Acupuncture ☐ Ice packs

Other: _____

Weather/ Altitude

Temperature: _____   Humidity: _____   Barometric pressure: _____

Pollen level: ☐ Low   ☐ Moderate   ☐ High   Current elevation: _____

Food Tracking

	Today	Yesterday
Meals/ snacks:		

	Today	Yesterday
Vitamins/ supplements:		

	Today	Past 5 days
Alcoholic beverages:		
Caffeinated beverages:		
8oz glasses of water:		

Additional Notes

_____

_____

_____

_____

_____

Doctor's Notes

Dr. Name: _____   Specialty: _____   Date: _____

_____

_____

_____

_____

_____

_____

Entry #: _____ Date: _____ Duration: _____

Onset: ☐ Slow ☐ Average ☐ Rapid

Pain level: ☐ Mild ☐ Moderate ☐ Severe

Pain Location
(Mark with an "X")

Pain Description

☐ Throbbing   ☐ Piercing   ☐ Pounding

☐ Dull   ☐ Burning   ☐ Pulsating

☐ Constant   ☐ Debilitating   ☐ Squeezing

☐ Other _____

Left, right, center: _____

Symptoms

☐ Light sensitivity   ☐ Sound sensitivity   ☐ Aura   ☐ Confusion

☐ Dizziness   ☐ Nausea   ☐ Vomiting   ☐ Chills

☐ Muscle aches   ☐ Muscle stiffness   ☐ Restlessness ☐ Congestion

☐ Coughing   ☐ Diarrhea   ☐ Fever   ☐ Sore throat

Other symptoms: _____

Health

Physical activity (past week):   ☐ Low   ☐ Moderate   ☐ High

Sleep quality (past week):   ☐ Poor ☐ Average   ☐ Good

Computer time (past week):   ☐ Low   ☐ Moderate   ☐ High

Stress level (past 3 days):   ☐ Low   ☐ Moderate   ☐ High

Hormones

☐ PMS   ☐ Menstruation   ☐ Menopause   ☐ Puberty   ☐ Other: _____

Treatments Applied

Medication(s)/
dosage: _____

☐ Massage   ☐ Stretching/ yoga   ☐ Nerve stimulation device

☐ Heat/bath   ☐ Acupuncture   ☐ Ice packs

Other: _____

Weather/ Altitude

Temperature: [   ]   Humidity: [   ]   Barometric pressure: [   ]

Pollen level: ☐ Low   ☐ Moderate   ☐ High   Current elevation: [   ]

Food Tracking

	Today	Yesterday
Meals/ snacks:		

	Today	Yesterday
Vitamins/ supplements:		

	Today	Past 5 days
Alcoholic beverages:		
Caffeinated beverages:		
8oz glasses of water:		

Additional Notes

_____
_____
_____
_____
_____

Doctor's Notes

Dr. Name: _____ Specialty: _____ Date: _____

_____
_____
_____
_____
_____
_____

Entry #: _____ Date: _____ Duration: _____

Onset: ☐ Slow ☐ Average ☐ Rapid

Pain level: ☐ Mild ☐ Moderate ☐ Severe

Pain Location
(Mark with an "X")

Pain Description

☐ Throbbing ☐ Piercing ☐ Pounding

☐ Dull ☐ Burning ☐ Pulsating

☐ Constant ☐ Debilitating ☐ Squeezing

☐ Other

Left, right, center:

Symptoms

☐ Light sensitivity ☐ Sound sensitivity ☐ Aura ☐ Confusion

☐ Dizziness ☐ Nausea ☐ Vomiting ☐ Chills

☐ Muscle aches ☐ Muscle stiffness ☐ Restlessness ☐ Congestion

☐ Coughing ☐ Diarrhea ☐ Fever ☐ Sore throat

Other symptoms:

Health

Physical activity (past week): ☐ Low ☐ Moderate ☐ High

Sleep quality (past week): ☐ Poor ☐ Average ☐ Good

Computer time (past week): ☐ Low ☐ Moderate ☐ High

Stress level (past 3 days): ☐ Low ☐ Moderate ☐ High

Hormones

☐ PMS ☐ Menstruation ☐ Menopause ☐ Puberty ☐ Other:

Treatments Applied

Medication(s)/ dosage:

☐ Massage ☐ Stretching/ yoga ☐ Nerve stimulation device

☐ Heat/bath ☐ Acupuncture ☐ Ice packs

Other:

Weather/ Altitude

Temperature: _____   Humidity: _____   Barometric pressure: _____

Pollen level: ☐ Low   ☐ Moderate   ☐ High   Current elevation: _____

Food Tracking

	Today	Yesterday
Meals/ snacks:		

	Today	Yesterday
Vitamins/ supplements:		

	Today	Past 5 days
Alcoholic beverages:		
Caffeinated beverages:		
8oz glasses of water:		

Additional Notes

_____

_____

_____

_____

_____

Doctor's Notes

Dr. Name: _____   Specialty: _____   Date: _____

_____

_____

_____

_____

_____

_____

Entry #: _____ Date: _____ Duration: _____

Onset: ☐ Slow ☐ Average ☐ Rapid

Pain level: ☐ Mild ☐ Moderate ☐ Severe

Pain Location
(Mark with an "X")

Left, right, center: _____

Pain Description

☐ Throbbing   ☐ Piercing   ☐ Pounding

☐ Dull   ☐ Burning   ☐ Pulsating

☐ Constant   ☐ Debilitating ☐ Squeezing

☐ Other _____

Symptoms

☐ Light sensitivity   ☐ Sound sensitivity   ☐ Aura   ☐ Confusion

☐ Dizziness   ☐ Nausea   ☐ Vomiting   ☐ Chills

☐ Muscle aches   ☐ Muscle stiffness   ☐ Restlessness ☐ Congestion

☐ Coughing   ☐ Diarrhea   ☐ Fever   ☐ Sore throat

Other symptoms: _____

Health

Physical activity (past week):   ☐ Low   ☐ Moderate   ☐ High

Sleep quality (past week):   ☐ Poor   ☐ Average   ☐ Good

Computer time (past week):   ☐ Low   ☐ Moderate   ☐ High

Stress level (past 3 days):   ☐ Low   ☐ Moderate   ☐ High

Hormones

☐ PMS   ☐ Menstruation   ☐ Menopause   ☐ Puberty   ☐ Other:

Treatments Applied

Medication(s)/ dosage: _____

☐ Massage   ☐ Stretching/ yoga   ☐ Nerve stimulation device

☐ Heat/bath   ☐ Acupuncture   ☐ Ice packs

Other: _____

Weather/ Altitude

Temperature: _____ Humidity: _____ Barometric pressure: _____

Pollen level: ☐ Low ☐ Moderate ☐ High Current elevation: _____

Food Tracking

	Today	Yesterday
Meals/ snacks:		

	Today	Yesterday
Vitamins/ supplements:		

	Today	Past 5 days
Alcoholic beverages:		
Caffeinated beverages:		
8oz glasses of water:		

Additional Notes

_____
_____
_____
_____
_____

Doctor's Notes

Dr. Name: _____ Specialty: _____ Date: _____

_____
_____
_____
_____
_____
_____

Entry #: _____ Date: _____ Duration: _____

Onset: ☐ Slow ☐ Average ☐ Rapid

Pain level: ☐ Mild ☐ Moderate ☐ Severe

Pain Location
(Mark with an "X")

Pain Description

☐ Throbbing ☐ Piercing ☐ Pounding

☐ Dull ☐ Burning ☐ Pulsating

☐ Constant ☐ Debilitating ☐ Squeezing

☐ Other _____

Left, right, center: _____

Symptoms

☐ Light sensitivity ☐ Sound sensitivity ☐ Aura ☐ Confusion

☐ Dizziness ☐ Nausea ☐ Vomiting ☐ Chills

☐ Muscle aches ☐ Muscle stiffness ☐ Restlessness ☐ Congestion

☐ Coughing ☐ Diarrhea ☐ Fever ☐ Sore throat

Other symptoms: _____

Health

Physical activity (past week): ☐ Low ☐ Moderate ☐ High

Sleep quality (past week): ☐ Poor ☐ Average ☐ Good

Computer time (past week): ☐ Low ☐ Moderate ☐ High

Stress level (past 3 days): ☐ Low ☐ Moderate ☐ High

Hormones

☐ PMS ☐ Menstruation ☐ Menopause ☐ Puberty ☐ Other: _____

Treatments Applied

Medication(s)/ dosage: _____

☐ Massage ☐ Stretching/ yoga ☐ Nerve stimulation device

☐ Heat/bath ☐ Acupuncture ☐ Ice packs

Other: _____

Weather/ Altitude

Temperature: _____ Humidity: _____ Barometric pressure:

Pollen level: ☐ Low ☐ Moderate ☐ High Current elevation: _____

Food Tracking

	Today	Yesterday
Meals/ snacks:		

	Today	Yesterday
Vitamins/ supplements:		

	Today	Past 5 days
Alcoholic beverages:		
Caffeinated beverages:		
8oz glasses of water:		

Additional Notes

_____
_____
_____
_____
_____

Doctor's Notes

Dr. Name: _____ Specialty: _____ Date: _____

_____
_____
_____
_____
_____
_____

Entry #: _____ Date: _____ Duration: _____

Onset: ☐ Slow ☐ Average ☐ Rapid

Pain level: ☐ Mild ☐ Moderate ☐ Severe

Pain Location
(Mark with an "X")

Pain Description

☐ Throbbing ☐ Piercing ☐ Pounding

☐ Dull ☐ Burning ☐ Pulsating

☐ Constant ☐ Debilitating ☐ Squeezing

☐ Other _____

Left, right, center: _____

Symptoms

☐ Light sensitivity ☐ Sound sensitivity ☐ Aura ☐ Confusion

☐ Dizziness ☐ Nausea ☐ Vomiting ☐ Chills

☐ Muscle aches ☐ Muscle stiffness ☐ Restlessness ☐ Congestion

☐ Coughing ☐ Diarrhea ☐ Fever ☐ Sore throat

Other symptoms: _____

Health

Physical activity (past week): ☐ Low ☐ Moderate ☐ High

Sleep quality (past week): ☐ Poor ☐ Average ☐ Good

Computer time (past week): ☐ Low ☐ Moderate ☐ High

Stress level (past 3 days): ☐ Low ☐ Moderate ☐ High

Hormones

☐ PMS ☐ Menstruation ☐ Menopause ☐ Puberty ☐ Other: _____

Treatments Applied

Medication(s)/dosage: _____

☐ Massage ☐ Stretching/ yoga ☐ Nerve stimulation device

☐ Heat/bath ☐ Acupuncture ☐ Ice packs

Other: _____

Weather/ Altitude

Temperature: _____   Humidity: _____   Barometric pressure: _____

Pollen level: ☐ Low   ☐ Moderate   ☐ High   Current elevation: _____

Food Tracking

	Today	Yesterday
Meals/ snacks:		

	Today	Yesterday
Vitamins/ supplements:		

	Today	Past 5 days
Alcoholic beverages:		
Caffeinated beverages:		
8oz glasses of water:		

Additional Notes

_____
_____
_____
_____
_____

Doctor's Notes

Dr. Name: _____   Specialty: _____   Date: _____

_____
_____
_____
_____
_____
_____

Entry #: _____ Date: _____ Duration: _____

Onset: ☐ Slow ☐ Average ☐ Rapid

Pain level: ☐ Mild ☐ Moderate ☐ Severe

Pain Location
(Mark with an "X")

Pain Description

☐ Throbbing ☐ Piercing ☐ Pounding

☐ Dull ☐ Burning ☐ Pulsating

☐ Constant ☐ Debilitating ☐ Squeezing

☐ Other _____

Left, right, center: _____

Symptoms

☐ Light sensitivity ☐ Sound sensitivity ☐ Aura ☐ Confusion

☐ Dizziness ☐ Nausea ☐ Vomiting ☐ Chills

☐ Muscle aches ☐ Muscle stiffness ☐ Restlessness ☐ Congestion

☐ Coughing ☐ Diarrhea ☐ Fever ☐ Sore throat

Other symptoms: _____

Health

Physical activity (past week): ☐ Low ☐ Moderate ☐ High

Sleep quality (past week): ☐ Poor ☐ Average ☐ Good

Computer time (past week): ☐ Low ☐ Moderate ☐ High

Stress level (past 3 days): ☐ Low ☐ Moderate ☐ High

Hormones

☐ PMS ☐ Menstruation ☐ Menopause ☐ Puberty ☐ Other: _____

Treatments Applied

Medication(s)/ dosage: _____

☐ Massage ☐ Stretching/ yoga ☐ Nerve stimulation device

☐ Heat/bath ☐ Acupuncture ☐ Ice packs

Other: _____

Weather/ Altitude

Temperature: _____ Humidity: _____ Barometric pressure: _____

Pollen level: ☐ Low ☐ Moderate ☐ High Current elevation: _____

Food Tracking

	Today	Yesterday
Meals/ snacks:		

	Today	Yesterday
Vitamins/ supplements:		

	Today	Past 5 days
Alcoholic beverages:		
Caffeinated beverages:		
8oz glasses of water:		

Additional Notes

_____
_____
_____
_____
_____

Doctor's Notes

Dr. Name: _____ Specialty: _____ Date: _____

_____
_____
_____
_____
_____
_____

Notes

Notes

Notes

Notes

Notes

Notes

Notes

Notes

Notes

Notes

Notes

Notes

Made in United States
Orlando, FL
26 September 2023

37294242R00078